AJPH
A PUBLICATION OF THE
AMERICAN PUBLIC HEALTH ASSOCIATION

AMERICAN JOURNAL of PUBLIC HEALTH
APRIL 2023
Issue 4

BUILDING BROAD PUBLIC HEALTH COALITIONS IN THE POST-*ROE* WORLD

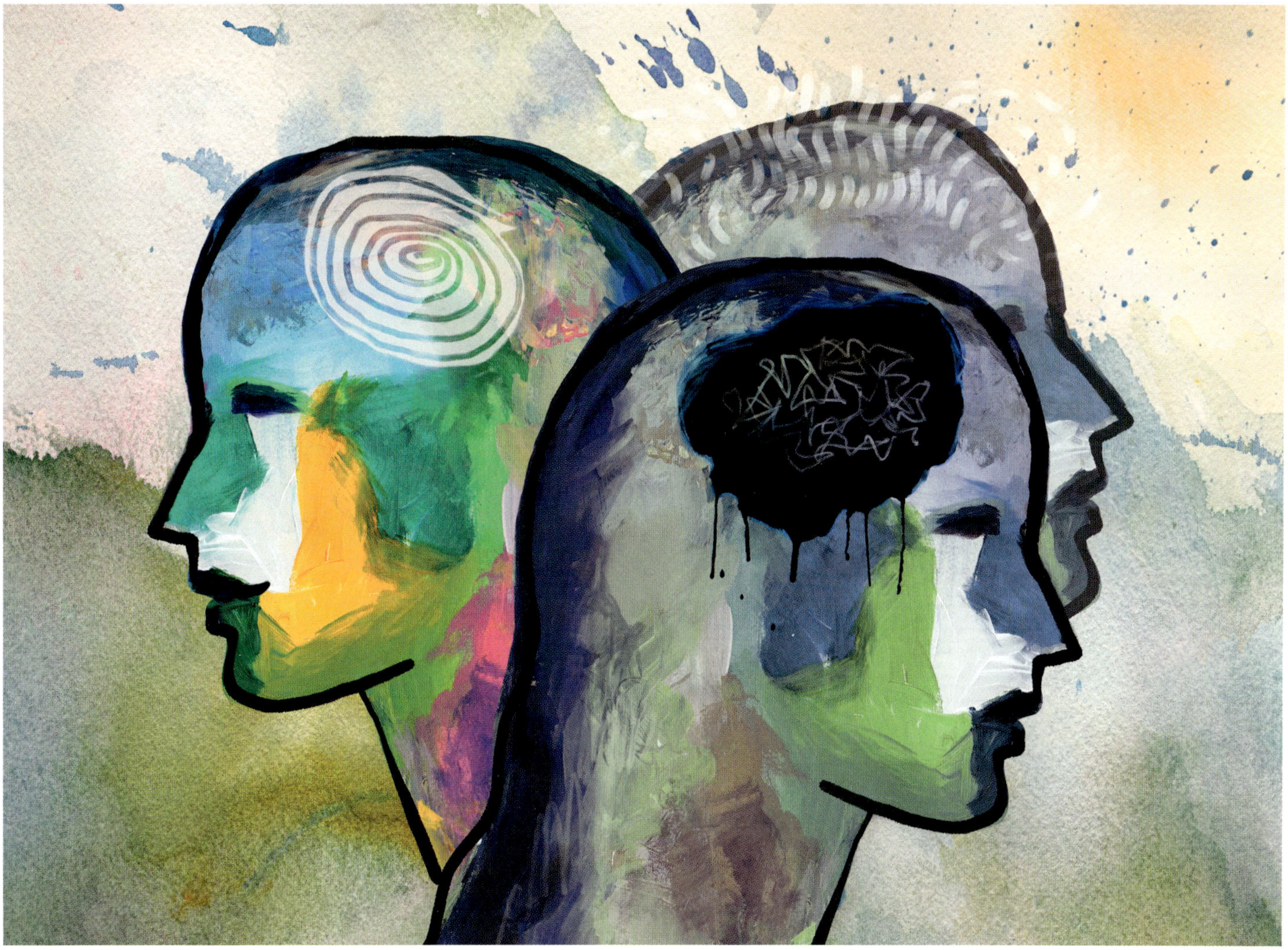

Common Ground on Abortion Rights, pp. 378 and 380

Mental and Physical Dangers, p. 382

Reproductive Health Care Physicians, p. 384

Codifying Abortion Rights, p. 386

A Dire State Context, p. 388

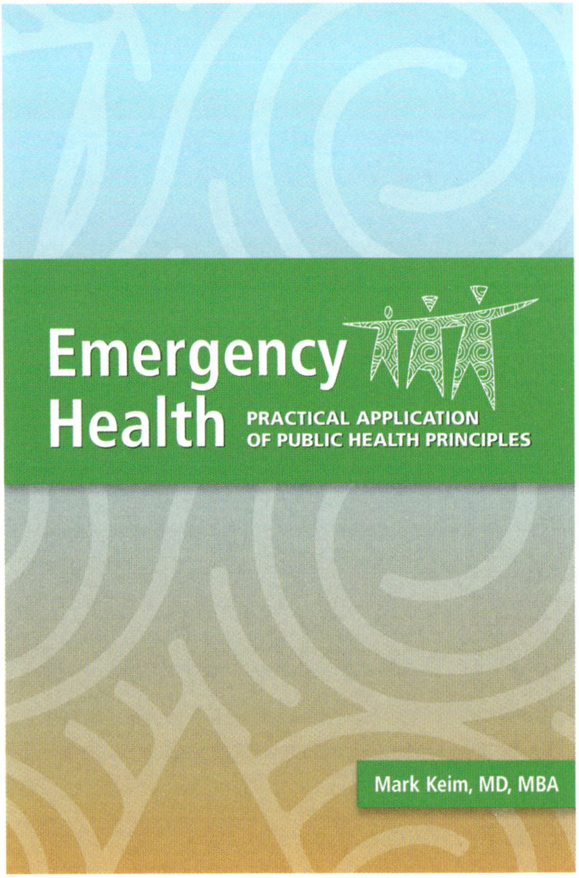

Emergency Health: Practical Application of Public Health Principles

By: Mark Keim, MD, MBA

978-0-87553-334-6, 336 PP, SOFTCOVER AND EBOOK, 2023

Emergency Health discusses the combination of disease prevention, health promotion and protection, and the provision of care related to disasters. This book stresses the importance of prioritizing equitable access to health before, during and after public health emergencies. It also examines public health's role in advocating for and implementing practices that reduce the impact of disasters on the larger ecosystem, thus benefiting health, wellness and health equity overall.

APHABOOKSTORE.ORG

APHA PRESS

AN IMPRINT OF AMERICAN PUBLIC HEALTH ASSOCIATION

APHA
AMERICAN PUBLIC HEALTH ASSOCIATION
For science. For action. For health.

AJPH®, published monthly, is the official Journal of the American Public Health Association®, 800 I St NW, Washington, DC 20001-3710; (202) 777- APHA; TDD (202) 777-2500. APHA is a nongovernmental professional society founded in 1872, representing all disciplines and specialties in public health.

The *American Journal of Public Health*® (*AJPH*) (print ISSN: 0090-0036; electronic ISSN: 1541- 0048), first published in 1911, is the official journal of the American Public Health Association® (APHA). The oldest and largest organization of public health professionals in the world, APHA represents approximately 30 000 members from more than 50 occupations of public health.

Submissions: Visit www.editorialmanager.com/ajph or ajph.edmgr.com for online manuscript preparation and submission guidelines. Contributions of original unpublished research, social science analyses, scholarly essays, critical commentaries, departments, and letters to the editor are welcome. Questions? Write ajph.submissions@apha.org or call APHA at (202) 777-2469.

Print plus online subscriptions: Institutional price (print copy with online access for a single institution and all authorized users, regardless of geographic location) varies by size of organization and ranges from $993–$1445 for US organizations, and $1073–$1526 for international organizations (air delivery); multiple campuses not permitted without special arrangement. Details of the tiered pricing system at https://subscriptionoffice.com/pages/apha-landing-page. To order, write apha.subscriptions@apha.org.

Online only subscriptions: Institutional price for one institution and its authorized users (regardless of geographic location) is $878–$1307. To order, write apha.subscriptions@apha.org. For academic consortia or multisite corporate subscriptions, contact apha.subscriptions@apha.org.

Print-only subscriptions: Institutional price is US $701, $782 international.

Back print issues: A limited number of print issues are for sale. Single copies are US $49, $55 international (air delivery). Shipping included; prepay only. To order, write apha.subscriptions@apha.org.

Reprints: For prices and ordering information on 50 or more reprints, check the Reprints section at www.ajph.org. To order smaller quantities of reprints (rush delivery), use the "Purchase Article" link on the article site itself.

Electronic access: Online articles more than 10 years old are available free for personal use at www.ajph.org. Recent articles are available through pay-per-view: single PDF article for $24, single issue access for 24 hours for $33, or entire site access for 24 hours for $38.

Postal information: Periodicals postage paid at Washington, DC, and additional mailing offices. Postmaster: Send address changes to American Journal of Public Health, 800 I St NW, Washington, DC 20001-3710.

Address changes: Send to AJPH, Membership Department (members) or AJPH Subscriptions (subscribers), APHA, 800 I St NW, Washington, DC 20001-3710. Or write to membership.mail@apha. org (members) or apha.subscriptions@apha.org (subscribers).

Advertising: For pricing and other information, see www.ajph.org. Please write to ashell.alston@ apha.org or call (202) 777-2470 for other advertising opportunities. Ask about special exhibit packages and sponsorships. Acceptance of advertising by the *Journal* does not imply endorsement of products.

Indexes: Publications that index or abstract articles from AJPH include the following: Ageline, Assia (Applied Social Science Index and Abstracts), Biological Abstracts, Chemical Abstracts, CINAHL, Criminal Justice Abstracts, EMBASE, EMCare, Environmental Abstracts, e-psyche, ERIC, ETOH (Alcohol and Alcohol Problems Science Database), Excerpta Medica, Food Science and Technology, General Science Index, Grateful Med, Hospital Literature Index, Human Resources Abstracts, International Pharmaceutical Abstracts (IPA), Medline, Physical Education Index, Pollution Abstracts, Psychological Abstracts, PsychINFO, Safety Science Abstracts, Sage Family Studies Abstracts, Sage Human Resources Abstracts, Science Citation Index, SCOPUS, SIIC Data Bases, Social Work Research and Abstracts, and Statistical Reference Index (SRI)/LexisNexis.

Medscape Publishers' Circle

AJPH

A PUBLICATION OF THE
AMERICAN PUBLIC HEALTH ASSOCIATION

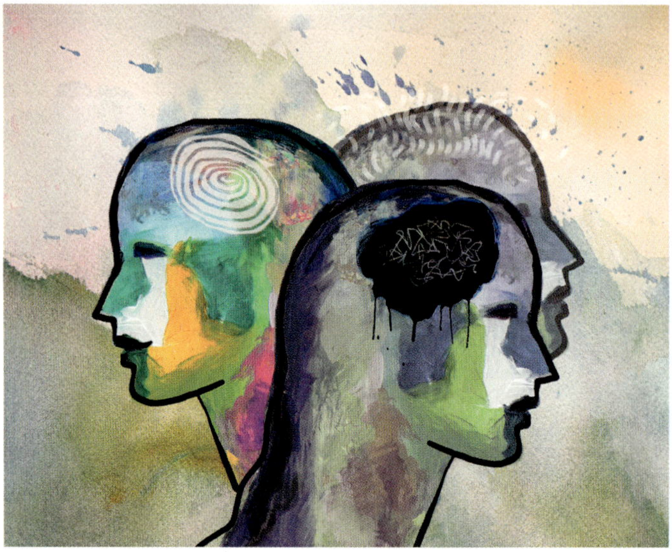

COVER: Navigating the fog for a clear view of health equity.

Cover concept and selection by Aleisha Kropf. Image by Stella Levi/Getty. Printed with permission.

APHA
AMERICAN PUBLIC HEALTH ASSOCIATION
For science. For action. For health.

Promoting public health research, policy, practice, and education is the *AJPH* mission. As we widen our scope to embrace global issues, we also sharpen our focus to support the needs of public health practitioners. We invite contributions of original unpublished research, opinion and commentary, and letters to the editor.

The *Journal* is printed on acid-free recycled paper.

OPEN ACCESS ONLINE ONLY PODCAST DATA SUPPLEMENT AVAILABLE

EDITOR'S CHOICE

349 Republicans Die More From COVID-19: Why We Care
A. Morabia

OPINIONS, IDEAS, & PRACTICE

EDITORIALS

350 Minors' Rights to Access Sexual and Reproductive Health Care
B. J. Hill

353 Improving Unequal Food Access Requires Understanding and Addressing the Social Inequalities That Contribute to It
S. Bowen and A. Hardison-Moody

356 Home Owners' Loan Corporation Maps and Place-Based Injury Risks: A Complex History
S. F. Jacoby

359 Bringing an Equity Lens to Address the Evolving Overdose Crisis: A Public Health of Consequence, April 2023
F. Kapadia

PERSPECTIVES

361 Improving the US and Global Pandemic Response: Lessons From Cuba
S. Galea and P. C. Erwin

NOTES FROM THE FIELD

363 Identifying COVID-19 Vaccine Deserts and Ways to Reduce Them: A Digital Tool to Support Public Health Decision-Making
R. L. Weintraub, K. Miller, B. Rader, J. Rosenberg, S. Srinath, S. R. Woodbury, M. D. Schultheiss, M. Kansal, S. Vispute, S. Serghiou, G. Flores, A. Kumok, T. Shekel, E. Gabrilovich, I. Ahmad, M. E. Chiang, and J. S. Brownstein

368 Improving Early Childhood Caries for American Indian 3- to 5-Year-Old Children Through Interprofessional Outreach: 2018–2022
L. S. Larsson and C. Hodgson

372 Statewide Policy to Increase Provision of Take-Home Naloxone at Emergency Department Visits for Opioid Overdose, Rhode Island, 2018–2019
J. Griffith, R. R. Yorlets, L. C. Chambers, C. S. Davis, A. Wentz, F. L. Beaudoin, J. Baird, and E. A. Samuels

REPRODUCTIVE RIGHTS AT THE STATE AND LOCAL LEVELS

378 Building Broad Public Health Coalitions in the Post-*Roe* World
A. Morabia

380 The Potential and Challenges for Common Ground on Abortion
S. Magnan

382 Denying Abortions Endangers Women's Mental and Physical Health
F. C. Worrell

384 Abortion Restrictions Threaten All Reproductive Health Care Clinicians
K. Brandi and P. Gill

386 Codify Abortion Rights and Access by Way of State Legislatures
D. Robinson and M. Simmons

388 Implications of *Dobbs v Jackson Women's Health Organization*
H. Palacio

RESEARCH & ANALYSIS

HISTORY

390 The First Publication on Contraception in a US Medical Journal, 1928: Hannah Mayer Stone's Case for Contraceptive Care Before the Pill
R. E. Jensen

LAW & ETHICS

397 Minor Consent Laws for Sexually Transmitted Infection and Human Immunodeficiency Virus Services in the United States: A Comprehensive, Longitudinal Survey of US State Laws
K. M. Nelson, A. Skinner, C. D. Stout, W. Raderman, E. Unger, J. Raifman, M. Agénor, M. L. Ybarra, S. I. Dunsiger, S. B. Austin, and K. Underhill

SURVEILLANCE

408 Overview of the 2019 National Health Interview Survey Questionnaire Redesign
B. Zablotsky, S. E. Lessem, R. M. Gindi, A. K. Maitland, J. M. Dahlhamer, and S. J. Blumberg

416 Methamphetamine-Related Mortality in the United States: Co-Involvement of Heroin and Fentanyl, 1999–2021
R. A. Hoopsick and R. A. Yockey

OPEN-THEMED RESEARCH

420 Structural Racism and Pedestrian Safety: Measuring the Association Between Historical Redlining and Contemporary Pedestrian Fatalities Across the United States, 2010–2019
N. L. Taylor, J. M. Porter, S. Bryan, K. J. Harmon, and L. S. Sandt

429 Abortion-Related Laws and Concurrent Patterns in Abortion Incidence in Indiana, 2010–2019
H. Moseson, M. H. Smith, P. Chakraborty, H. J. Gyuras, A. Foster, D. Bessett, T. A. Wilkinson, and A. H. Norris

438 Impact of School Shootings on Adolescent School Safety, 2009–2019
J. C. Hodges, D. T. Walker, C. F. Baum, and S. S. Hawkins

442 Housing Instability and Evictions Linked to Elevated Intimate Partner and Workplace Violence Among Women Sex Workers in Vancouver, Canada: Findings of a Prospective, Community-Based Cohort, 2010–2019
S. M. Goldenberg, N. Buglioni, A. Krüsi, E. Frost, S. Moreheart, M. Braschel, and K. Shannon

BACKMATTER

OTHER DEPARTMENTS

456 Subscription Form

Republicans Die More From COVID-19: Why We Care

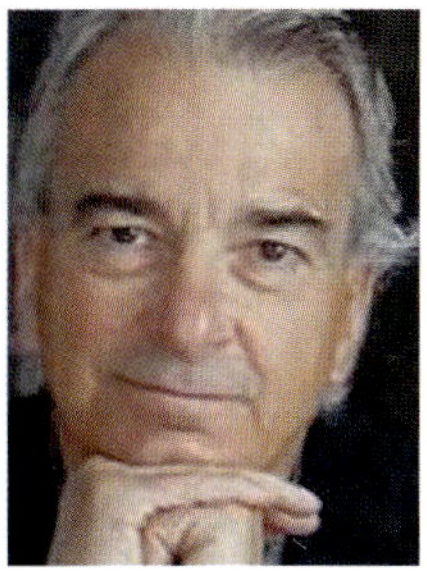

In a September 2022 study from the National Bureau of Economic Research (NBER), in Cambridge, Massachusetts (http://www.nber.org/papers/w30512), Wallace et al. compared the excess mortality among Republicans and Democrats from 2018 to 2022. Excess deaths during the pandemic were computed relative to the number of deaths observed in 2019. There was no difference in excess deaths along partisan lines in 2018, indicating that the two groups were comparable. However, since the introduction of COVID-19 vaccines, the excess death rate among Republicans was 10.4 percentage points higher than among Democrats, or 1.5 times that of the Democrats.

If 234 000 deaths from COVID-19 could have been prevented with a primary series of vaccinations (https://bit.ly/3XrFXfz) between June 2021 and March 2022, I estimate that 140 400 of these deaths would have been among Republicans. This is, of course, not a surprise because Republicans are less likely to be vaccinated than Democrats, and, as the Texas Department of Health put it, "Texas Data Shows Unvaccinated People 20 times More Likely to Die From COVID-19" (https://bit.ly/3H0ACog). The Republicans die at higher rates than Democrats mostly in counties with low vaccination rates.

This is not a study based on county-level statistics, which are often tricky to interpret in terms of causal relation. The authors have linked individual-level information both on mortality from 2018 to 2021 and on political affiliation from 2017 voter registration in Ohio and Florida.

In the current state of tension between the most vocal and extremist faction of the Republican party and Democrats, some people may think: if COVID-19 kills Republicans, why should we care? The answer is very clear. Such reasoning is incompatible with the public health approach. Public health needs to be all-inclusive to succeed. Viruses do not sense political affiliation. The overmortality among Republicans stems from sectors of the population being unvaccinated. This has translated into a longer duration of the pandemic, more new variants, more deaths, more school closures, small businesses filing for bankruptcy, and misery for everyone. The response to a public health emergency is either successfully collective, or it fails. A striking finding of the NBER study is that in the counties with at least 50% of the population vaccinated, there were no excess death differences between Republicans and Democrats. The vaccinated protected the unvaccinated.

There are three reasons why some Americans may not have been vaccinated. The first and most important one is that some people may want to be vaccinated and do not have access to the intervention. This is the main challenge for public health. It is also the main reason why protecting the community involves using the force of the law when needed to implement a public health mandate. Most Americans got the point that vaccines are a collective response to a collective threat and that the mandates are also the optimal solution for individuals. They voted with their arms.

A second reason for not being vaccinated comes from a misunderstanding about what public health is. Vaccines are different from a medical prescription that each of us is free to accept or refuse. They are prescribed for the whole community. Vaccinated persons protect those who are unvaccinated, and the unvaccinated put vaccinated persons at risk. The main and often only interface between Americans and the health sector is clinical medicine, not public health. The current pandemic is an opportunity to explain the difference between the individual approach of clinical medicine and the collective approach of public health. Both have the same goal: protecting each individual.

Finally, the third reason for not being vaccinated is to be opposed to it. The public health approach prioritizes trying to convince as much of the population as possible to follow public health recommendations. Making public health mandates the law enables reaching a political consensus that makes them enforceable. Few will disagree that today's employers should be punished if they employ minors in their warehouse, but the principle behind the 1938 Fair Labor Standards Act is the same as for a vaccine mandate, a collective defense of the right to health that no individual can wage alone.

So, yes, we should care about Republicans dying more than Democrats because of the COVID-19 pandemic. Public health is all-inclusive. It should be able to reach and protect everyone: Republicans, immigrants, the poor—everyone. AJPH

Alfredo Morabia, MD, PhD
AJPH *Editor-in-Chief*
@AlfredoMorabia

DOI: https://doi.org/10.2105/AJPH.2023.307237

30 Years Ago

Pennsylvania's Birth Rates After Medicaid Abortion Restrictions

The right to legal abortion was effectively terminated for many Pennsylvania women in 1985, when state lawmakers restricted Medicaid funding for abortion to pregnancies that are life-threatening or result from rape or incest. An examination of state health department statistics from 1980 through 1990 . . . reveals that, beginning in 1985, there was a marked increase in the ratio of live births to abortions. . . . During these years, live birth rates did not increase nationwide to the degree that they did in Pennsylvania and in other states with newly initiated Medicaid restrictions. Thus, one might reasonably infer that the change in Pennsylvania rates was due in large part to Medicaid-eligible women who, faced with unintended pregnancy, chose to give birth as the only affordable option. Because of the ramifications of poverty, the denial of Medicaid-funded abortion to poor women is likely to cause financial, emotional, and physical hardships even beyond those that would be experienced by more affluent women who for some reason were unable to get legal abortions. Thus, many of the babies born to these lower-income women must begin their lives with the risks of poverty compounded by the risks of unwantedness.

From AJPH, June 1993, pp. 911–912

52 Years Ago

Legal Authority of Health Departments to Regulate Abortion Practice

The first health department to take action to regulate abortion practice was in New York City which enacted amendments to its Health Code. . . . The New York City regulations are quite thorough and detailed. The greatest amount of publicity has been given to the prohibition of abortions in doctors' offices. All legal abortions in New York City under these regulations must be performed in an "abortion service." . . . It has been argued that prevention of abortions in doctors' offices forces the entire load on inadequate facilities in hospitals and clinics and that waiting lists will be dangerously long. This is a serious problem. However, it is aggravated in New York City by the fact that the population is so great and by large numbers of nonresidents coming to the city for abortions. It points up the fact that the change in the laws in this country on a state-by-state basis is a problem in itself, particularly on such matters as abortion.

From AJPH, March 1971, pp. 623 and 625

Minors' Rights to Access Sexual and Reproductive Health Care

B. Jessie Hill, JD

ABOUT THE AUTHOR

B. Jessie Hill is with the School of Law, Case Western Reserve University, Cleveland, OH.

See also Nelson et al., p. 397.

Young people face significant unaddressed health care needs in the United States. For example, as Nelson et al. explain in this issue of *AJPH*, adolescents—especially those who are already marginalized because of their racial, ethnic, sexual, or gender identity—are significantly affected by sexually transmitted infections (STIs) such as HIV (https://bit.ly/3jKUzYL). Yet, the law governing minors' access to sensitive health care services is a morass.[1] A sensible policy response, recognizing the basic human and constitutional right of mature minors to access health care without parental involvement, is urgently needed.

THE PATCHWORK OF MINOR CONSENT LAWS

Although individuals younger than the age of majority are generally deemed legally incapable of consenting to health care on their own, states have made numerous exceptions to this broad (and perhaps overstated) rule. Nelson et al. point out that all 50 states and the District of Columbia allow minors to seek testing and treatment of STIs without parental consent (https://bit.ly/3jKUzYL). In addition, many states allow minors to consent on their own to substance abuse treatment, mental health services (on an outpatient basis), examination and treatment for sexual assault, prenatal care, and contraceptive services.[1]

Numerous states permit minors deemed "mature" to consent to care as if they were adults. This includes "emancipated" minors who are living on their own and supporting themselves, as well as those mature minors who are found to have sufficient capacity to "appreciat[e] the nature, extent, and consequences" of the treatment and to "weigh the risks and benefits,"[2] as determined on a case-by-case basis (though some states have also established a minimum age for a minor to qualify as such). These pathways have their limitations, however; not all states recognize the so-called mature-minor doctrine, and even in those that do, a clinician may not feel comfortable providing care to a young person if that decision may later be second-guessed by an unhappy and litigious guardian.[3]

Moreover, even minors who are considered mature or emancipated are not always considered to have the same capacity as adults to make health care decisions. For example, in 1989, the Illinois Supreme Court found that a 17-year-old suffering from terminal leukemia was mature enough to refuse blood transfusions for religious reasons.[4] However, the court also held that, despite her maturity, the minor's decision would have to be weighed against the state's interests, such as in preserving life and maintaining the ethical integrity of the medical profession.

MINORS' HUMAN RIGHT TO REPRODUCTIVE AND SEXUAL HEALTH CARE

Access to health care, including sexual and reproductive health care, is a human right.[5] It should not be subject to a confusing patchwork of rules that obstructs some of the most vulnerable among us from achieving good health. Indeed, World Health Organization guidelines urge expanded access for adolescents to sexual and reproductive health care, in recognition of its importance "for the human rights, health and well-being of adolescents."[6(p1)]

Similarly, through the federal Title X program, which provides free or low-cost sexual and reproductive health care to adolescents as well as adults, the US government has recognized "that without access to confidential care, many adolescents would not seek needed health services."[7(p48)] However, Title X's confidentiality requirements apply only to clinics that receive Title X grants, and Nelson et al. point out that those clinics are not where the majority of adolescents access care (https://bit.ly/3jKUzYL). Minors should have the right to access all medically appropriate reproductive and sexual health care services—including treatment and testing for STIs and HIV, examination for and treatment of sexual assault, gender-affirming health care, prenatal care, contraceptive services, and abortion care—across the board without parental consent or notification, regardless of whether they access that care at a federally funded Title X site.

One possibility would be to adopt universally the approach that Title X currently takes, requiring parental participation when feasible but disclaiming any legal requirement of notice or consent. That rule states that family involvement should be encouraged "[t]o the extent practical," but also that "Title X projects may not require consent of parents or guardians for the provision of services to minors, nor . . . notify a parent or guardian before or after a minor has requested and/or received" family planning services.[8]

Another possibility would be a mature minor rule that applies nationwide. In the 1979 case *Bellotti v. Baird*, the US Supreme Court held that minors who are mature and well-informed must have a right to access abortion without parental consent.[9] The same is true for minors for whom the abortion would be in their best interests. Although the right identified in *Bellotti* has not been explicitly extended to other medical services, as *Bellotti* relied partly on the Court's recognition of a constitutional right to reproductive privacy, it is unclear why minors who are sufficiently mature, or for whom immediate treatment would be in their best interests, should not possess the same ability. While pregnant minors are in a somewhat unique situation in that they are facing a time-sensitive decision with potentially profound long-term effects on that young person's future, minors suffering from STIs, for example, are similarly positioned in terms of the gravity of their situations and the need for immediate treatment.

ATTACKS ON REPRODUCTIVE AND SEXUAL HEALTH CARE

As Nelson et al. demonstrate, the trend toward empowering minors to access health care without parental involvement steadily strengthened throughout the twentieth century, but it has recently plateaued (Figure 1 in Nelson et al., https://bit.ly/3jKUzYL). Unfortunately, the prospects for breaking through the plateau are grim. With the overruling of *Roe v. Wade* and the rise of controversies over minors' access to gender-affirming care, even with parental consent, minors' access to sensitive health care is increasingly threatened. The US Supreme Court's June 2022 ruling in *Dobbs v. Jackson Women's Health Organization* threw into question the basis for minors' constitutional rights to access abortion and contraception without parental consent, opening up the possibility of further attacks on minors' access to health care.[10] And several states, including Alabama, Arkansas, Florida, Tennessee, and Texas, have sought to take action against minors' access to trans health care, even when parents are involved in the care.[11]

Moreover, Title X has been under attack, as some groups have sought not only to push parental participation but also to hamstring Title X providers and prevent them from offering nondirective, comprehensive counseling. A rule that was briefly in effect during the Trump administration encouraged family participation in minors' care without emphasizing the need for confidentiality and included other requirements that, together, resulted in approximately one fifth of the clinics previously in the program leaving the program and, thus, a severe reduction in the program's capacity to serve all populations.[12]

The continuing harm to the health and human rights of young people in the United States is unjustifiable, especially given that policymakers have recognized the need for confidential access without parental involvement in some states and for some types of services. It is well past time to extend that right to all minors seeking confidential reproductive and sexual health services. AJPH

CORRESPONDENCE

Correspondence should be sent to B. Jessie Hill, Case Western Reserve University School of Law, 11075 East Boulevard, Cleveland, OH 44106 (e-mail: bjh11@case.edu). Reprints can be ordered at https://ajph.org by clicking the "Reprints" link.

PUBLICATION INFORMATION

Full Citation: Hill BJ. Minors' rights to access sexual and reproductive health care. *Am J Public Health*. 2023;113(4):350–352.

Acceptance Date: January 14, 2023.

DOI: https://doi.org/10.2105/AJPH.2023.307235

CONFLICTS OF INTEREST

The author has no conflicts of interest.

REFERENCES

1. Hill BJ. Medical decision making by and on behalf of adolescents: reconsidering first principles. *J Health Care Law Policy*. 2012;15(1):37–73.
2. *Cardwell v. Bechtol*, 724 SW2d 739 (Tenn 1987).
3. Benston S. Not of minor consequence?: Medical decision-making autonomy and the Mature Minor Doctrine. *Indiana Health Law Rev*. 2016;13(1):1–16. https://doi.org/10.18060/3911.0011
4. *In re E.G.*, 549 NE2d 322 (Ill 1989).
5. Gable L. Reproductive health as a human right. *Case West Reserve Law Rev*. 2010;60(4):957–996. https://doi.org/10.2139/SSRN.1865841
6. World Health Organization. WHO Recommendations on Adolescent Sexual and Reproductive Health and Rights. 2018. Available at: https://www.who.int/publications/i/item/9789241514606. Accessed January 28, 2023.
7. Hasstedt K. Ensuring adolescents' ability to obtain confidential family planning services in Title X. *Guttmacher Policy Rev*. 2018;21:48–54.
8. 45 CFR §59.10(b).
9. *Bellotti v. Baird*, 443 US 622 (1979).

10. *Dobbs v. Jackson Women's Health Org,* 142 S Ct 2228 (2022).
11. Fiore K. It's been a tough year for transgender medicine—hospitals have been threatened, scientific debate has been weaponized. *MedPage Today*. December 28, 2022. Available at: https://www.medpagetoday.com/special-reports/features/102408. Accessed January 28, 2023.
12. Dawson R. Trump administration's domestic gag rule has slashed the Title X network's capacity by half. Guttmacher Institute. February 2020. Available at: https://www.guttmacher.org/article/2020/02/trump-administrations-domestic-gag-rule-has-slashed-title-x-networks-capacity-half. Accessed January 28, 2023.

Improving Unequal Food Access Requires Understanding and Addressing the Social Inequalities That Contribute to It

Sarah Bowen, PhD, and Annie Hardison-Moody, PhD

ABOUT THE AUTHORS

Sarah Bowen is with the Department of Sociology and Anthropology, North Carolina State University, Raleigh. Annie Hardison-Moody is with the Department of Agricultural and Human Sciences, North Carolina State University.

The food landscape in rural communities is shifting. Dollar stores have moved in as grocery stores have closed. However, we still know little about whether and how this has altered people's food-shopping behaviors. In last month's issue of *AJPH*, Feng et al.[1] used a national data set of food expenditures to chart changes in food spending at different types of retail outlets between 2008 and 2020. They found that, over this period, dollar stores grew faster than any other type of food retailer in terms of share of food spending and that rural households' share outpaced that of other households.

The research by Feng et al. offers clear evidence of the need to consider dollar stores in conversations about improving food access, especially in rural areas. They also call for additional research on the implications for public health. We concur. Furthermore, we argue that improving unequal food access requires understanding and addressing the structural inequalities that contribute to it. We offer the following key considerations to ground this work.

First, it is important to recognize that rural areas are not a monolith. Rurality shapes food access in important ways, but food access also varies widely in rural areas. As Feng et al. show, rural Black households spend, by far, the largest share (11.6%) of their food budget at dollar stores, and the share of food spending at dollar stores is higher for rural households in the South. Similarly, many of the counties with the highest rates of food insecurity are rural Southern counties with large shares of people of color.[2] Structural racism, in the form of decades of disinvestment and discrimination, has shaped economic development and access to both social services and food in these communities.[3]

Second, to understand the implications of the increased reliance on dollar stores, we need to look more closely at how people are using them. As Feng et al. note, the stores themselves vary. Although many dollar stores carry only shelf-stable foods and beverages, others offer eggs, milk, and even fresh produce. We also know from previous research on food access that shopping patterns are complicated; people base their decisions on where to shop on a range of criteria, including proximity, price, and quality.[4,5] Understanding the particulars of food decisions requires paying attention to the stories and complexities of life for people in rural communities.

Between 2012 and 2020, we conducted four waves of semistructured interviews with 124 low-income female caregivers in North Carolina, including 85 rural households.[6] In one set of interviews, we asked caregivers to describe their shopping habits in detail. Although most people shopped primarily at supermarkets,[5] many—especially in the most rural county—also relied on dollar stores. Not surprisingly, proximity was important; people said that if they ran out of only one or two items, they would try to get it at the dollar store rather than going all the way to the supermarket (which was often much farther away). Many people also shopped at dollar stores purposefully as part of a strategy focused on feeding their families on very tight budgets. They discussed buying specific items at dollar stores—snacks, but also spices, canned goods, cereal, rice, bread, and even, participants told us, ground beef or frozen tilapia—because they were cheapest. Alyssa, a mother of three, said she went to the dollar store first to get sides and basics: "So I can see how much money I save before I go over [to the supermarket]." As Feng et al. point out, people make food decisions for complex reasons, and efforts to improve food access should start by recognizing this.

AJPH April 2023, Vol 113, No. 4

Third, it is important to consider how dollar stores affect communities. On one hand, dollar stores can serve as community assets as affordable and local options for buying food.[7] On the other hand, they also can displace local businesses and often fail to offer healthy options such as fresh produce.[8,9] Improving dollar stores' offerings requires understanding them as part of communities. Some of the caregivers in our study worked in dollar stores or had friends or relatives who worked in them. They talked about going to (or avoiding) specific stores because the employees were helpful or made them feel welcome (or, conversely, made them feel unwelcome). Dollar stores' offerings also vary. Although previous research clearly shows that they offer fewer healthy items than supermarkets,[8] some in our study were better than others (offering fresh meat or fish, for example, or frozen vegetables).

We also saw examples of how communities are partnering with dollar stores to improve food access. In one of the rural counties in our study, a family and consumer science agent connected local farmers who wished to sell their produce at dollar and corner stores in an effort to support local agriculture and make healthy, convenient snacks available to consumers. Anecdotes like these, although rare, demonstrate how community members need to be at the center of conversations about the impacts of dollar stores on the places where they live.[10]

Finally, we want to underscore what other researchers have also argued: food access is, most fundamentally, about money. It is important that people have access to stores offering the foods they need at prices they can afford. However, the most critical step for improving food access is addressing the systemic inequities that leave people without adequate economic resources. During the COVID-19 pandemic, various social support programs were created or expanded, providing a natural experiment on how increasing social support improves people's access to food. Using repeated surveys of a nationally representative sample of US households, Shafer et al. showed how the introduction of advance payments for the Child Tax Credit was associated with a 26% reduction in household food insufficiency.[11] When the payments expired, food insufficiency increased.[12]

We conducted a qualitative study of experiences of food insecurity during the pandemic, interviewing families in rural and urban counties in five states (Michigan, Mississippi, North Carolina, South Carolina, and South Dakota).[13] People told us that programs like the expansion of SNAP (the Supplemental Nutrition Assistance Program), stimulus checks, and the Child Tax Credit had allowed them to stock up on key freezer and nonperishable foods, sometimes for the first time in years, providing an important buffer against future food insecurity.

In closing, the analysis by Feng et al. offers an important glimpse into how food purchases are shifting in rural US communities. As public health researchers and practitioners seek to understand why these changes are happening and how they matter, it is critical to center the lives and histories of the people and communities who are most affected by these changes. We must use a food justice lens to improve food access, seeking to understand where inequities exist and who is affected, as well as how community members and leaders are responding. AJPH

CORRESPONDENCE

Correspondence should be sent to Sarah Bowen, Campus Box 8107, Raleigh, NC 27695 (e-mail: sarah_bowen@ncsu.edu). Reprints can be ordered at http://www.ajph.org by clicking the "Reprints" link.

PUBLICATION INFORMATION

Full Citation: Bowen S, Hardison-Moody A. Improving unequal food access requires understanding and addressing the social inequalities that contribute to it. *Am J Public Health.* 2023;113(4):353–355.

Acceptance Date: January 21, 2023.

DOI: https://doi.org/10.2105/AJPH.2023.307243

CONTRIBUTORS

Both authors participated in the conceptualization and writing of the editorial and in the research project mentioned in the editorial.

ACKNOWLEDGMENTS

Research discussed in this editorial was supported by the US Department of Agriculture, National Institute of Food and Agriculture (grant 2011-68001-30103), the Russell Sage Foundation (grant G-1902-11562), and the National Science Foundation (grant 2032563).

Note. All the opinions, findings, and recommendations expressed here are those of the authors and do not necessarily reflect the views of the funders.

CONFLICTS OF INTEREST

The authors have no conflicts of interest to disclose.

REFERENCES

1. Feng W, Page ET, Cash SB. Dollar stores and food access for rural households in the United States, 2008–2020. *Am J Public Health.* 2023; 113(3):331–340.
2. Hake M, Engelhard E, Dewey A. Map the meal gap 2022: a report on county and congressional district food insecurity and county food cost in the United States in 2020. July 2022. Available at: https://www.feedingamerica.org/sites/default/files/2022-09/Map%20the%20Meal%20Gap%202022%20Report_0.pdf. Accessed January 24, 2023.
3. Bowen S, Elliott S, Hardison-Moody A. The structural roots of food insecurity: how racism is a fundamental cause of food insecurity. *Sociol Compass.* 2021;15(7):e12846. https://doi.org/10.1111/soc4.12846
4. Cannuscio CC, Tappe K, Hillier A, Buttenheim A, Karpyn A, Glanz K. Urban food environments and residents' shopping behaviors. *Am J Prev Med.* 2013;45(5):606–614. https://doi.org/10.1016/j.amepre.2013.06.021
5. MacNell L. A geo-ethnographic analysis of low-income rural and urban women's food shopping behaviors. *Appetite.* 2018;128:311–320. https://doi.org/10.1016/j.appet.2018.05.147
6. Bowen S, Elliott S, Hardison-Moody A. Rural food insecurity: a longitudinal analysis of low-income

rural households with children in the South. *RSF.* 2022;8(3):50–77. https://doi.org/10.7758/RSF.2022.8.3.02

7. Coughenour C, Bungum TJ, Regalado MN. Healthy food options at dollar discount stores are equivalent in quality and lower in price compared to grocery stores: an examination in Las Vegas, NV. *Int J Environ Res Public Health.* 2018;15(12):2773. https://doi.org/10.3390/ijerph15122773
8. Caspi CE, Pelletier JE, Harnack L, Erickson DJ, Laska MN. Differences in healthy food supply and stocking practices between small grocery stores, gas-marts, pharmacies and dollar stores. *Public Health Nutr.* 2016;19(3):540–547. https://doi.org/10.1017/S1368980015002724
9. Marchesi K, Lopez R, Steinbach S. Dollar store expansion, food retail competition, and rural employment. Paper presented at: Allied Social Sciences Association Annual Meeting, New Orleans, LA; January 6–8, 2023.
10. Greenfield N. From farms to dollar stores, one woman's fight for justice. August 23, 2019. Available at: https://www.nrdc.org/stories/farms-dollar-stores-one-womans-fight-justice. Accessed January 20, 2023.
11. Shafer PR, Gutiérrez KM, Ettinger de Cuba S, Bovell-Ammon A, Raifman J. Association of the implementation of child tax credit advance payments with food insufficiency in US households. *JAMA Netw Open.* 2022;5(1):e2143296. https://doi.org/10.1001/jamanetworkopen.2021.43296
12. Bovell-Ammon A, McCann NC, Mulugeta M, Ettinger de Cuba S, Raifman J, Shafer P. Association of the expiration of child tax credit advance payments with food insufficiency in US households. *JAMA Netw Open.* 2022;5(10):e2234438. https://doi.org/10.1001/jamanetworkopen.2022.34438
13. Bowen S, Hardison-Moody A, Eshleman K, et al. The impact of COVID-19 on experiences of food insecurity across place: a qualitative research protocol. *Int J Qual Methods.* 2021;20. https://doi.org/10.1177/16094069211062416

Home Owners' Loan Corporation Maps and Place-Based Injury Risks: A Complex History

Sara F. Jacoby, PhD, MSN, MPH

ABOUT THE AUTHOR

Sara F. Jacoby is with the School of Nursing, University of Pennsylvania, Philadelphia.

See also Taylor et al., p. 420.

AJPH April 2023, Vol 113, No. 4

In a piece for *Ebony* magazine in 1965, James Baldwin made a statement now inscribed on a wall at the National Museum of African American History and Culture that "the great force of history comes from the fact that we carry it within us . . . history is literally present in all that we do."[1(p.47)] Historical context shapes the ways in which individuals embody the circumstances to which they are born and in which they live.[2] It is the backdrop for every public health problem and all that public health data can enumerate.

The historical context of the United States is inseparable from its history of racism and of the institutions and policies that reify racialized economic segregation and social inequality.[3] Let us consider the public health problem of physical injuries as a leading cause of death and disability across the life span.[4] There are persistent population-level disparities in injury risks and outcomes associated with race, ethnicity, economic resources, and geography.[4] Treating these disparities as ahistorical phenomena has some advantages for simple, structural public health interventions. However, viewing any health disparity through a solely contemporary lens may obscure critical opportunities for intervention that require appreciation for how injury risks and outcomes have been racialized and emplaced across US geography.

LINKING REDLINING AND PEDESTRIAN INJURIES

Following the digital publication of the University of Richmond's Mapping Inequality project,[5] there has been a notable increase in research attempting to link historical structural racism in the housing market to the contemporary distribution of fatal and nonfatal injuries. In their article in this issue of *AJPH*, Taylor et al. (p. 420) add to this area of work. They overlay mortality data from the Fatality Analysis Reporting System of the National Highway Traffic Safety Administration onto digitized renderings of more than 200 Home Owners' Loan Corporation (HOLC) security maps from across US metropolitan areas. Taylor et al. tested their proposition that historical structural racism in the housing market created the conditions for lower-income communities and communities of color to experience higher risks for pedestrian injuries today. Structural racism, in this study, was operationalized as the grading of the geography depicted in HOLC maps from which the term redlining is derived. They found statistically significant associations between the spatial distribution of pedestrian fatalities in the past decade and HOLC grading schemas created in the 1930s.

Taylor et al. make clear that operationalizing structural racism through HOLC maps creates important limitations in the interpretation of their findings. They discuss why HOLC maps offer a limited view of structural racism as defined in Bailey et al. as "mutually reinforcing systems of housing, education, employment, earnings, benefits, credit, media, health care, and criminal justice . . . [that] reinforce discriminatory beliefs, values, and the distribution of resources."[6(p.1545)] What is missing from this discussion is that HOLC grading schemas when aggregated at the national level can conceal how structural racism plays out within local context and local change over time. In some places, HOLC maps may be an artifact of discriminatory thought at a specific and limited point in history, and in others they will have had a direct contributory role in the perpetuation of discrimination in the private housing market.[7]

LIMITATIONS OF INTERPRETATION

Hillier determined substantial inconsistencies between grades on HOLC maps and actual mortgage lending practices using the history of the city of Philadelphia as an example.[8] Many HOLC maps are likely misrepresentations. This should prompt additional pause when interpreting this current analysis within the growing body of work that uses HOLC spatial data to represent the processes that forged racialized economic segregation and their impact on present-day injury outcomes.

Historian Robert Gioielli emphasizes that while maps can be powerful models for health communication, as sources of data they can "flatten and simplify complex stories."[7] He describes the ways in which HOLC maps were just one manifestation of forms of racism that shaped the history of the US housing market. There were discriminatory policies and practices that existed before the creation of HOLC maps, and there are discriminatory policies and practices after their creation that maintain racial and economic inequality in the marketing of private property and its ownership. Focusing on the direct statistical association between HOLC map grading and public health outcomes, he maintains, overattributes determinants of health to long-gone actors and institutions. This kind of interpretation lets society too easily "off the hook" for the ways in which structural racism plays out through contemporary actions and institutions.

Beyond interpretative limitations, Taylor et al. discuss the methodological challenge they encountered when linking historical spatial data at a census tract level to data from the US Census's American Community Survey and injury fatality registries. Noelke et al. determined that when comparing HOLC area boundaries to the present distribution of various health outcomes at the census tract level, there is an array of analytic choices that can affect model performance.[9] They found that while there are opportunities to optimize models, most previously used approaches perform more or less similarly in their ability to predict health outcomes. Without concerted effort, even the most optimized models will not address the influence of intermediary and intermediate forms of structural racism in housing market on pedestrian injury risks and mortality.

CONTEXT FOR INTERVENTION

Graetz and Esposito advance the work of connecting historical HOLC maps to the distribution of health outcomes through causal mediation analyses. They tested the relationship between life expectancy and racialized public–private investment, valuation of place, steering in the real estate market, and economic inequality.[10] They found that HOLC area grades predict only a small proportion of total disparity between contemporary Black and White life expectancy and concluded that redlining should not be interpreted as a point-in-time exposure but, rather, as a series of processes and relationships embedded in the distribution of proximate influences on place-based health.

Future public health injury research will ideally address more complex interpretations of the ways in which injury outcomes are impacted by structural racism in the housing market. The field would likely benefit from collaboration with historians and other social scientists who can deepen the nuance of approaches used when modeling data and when deriving meaning from model outcomes. But despite interpretive and methodologic limitations, the work by Taylor et al. is important as a new perspective on the trajectory between historical racism and inequities in transportation and traffic safety. Their results reinforce other studies indicating a statistically supported association between HOLC area grading and injury-related morbidity and mortality. Taylor et al. conclude that, in addition to prompting more research, their findings indicate that public health safety interventions should focus on modifying the underlying causes of political, social, and built environmental inequities. In other words, it may well be time to use this kind of research evidence to inform the extent of resources and infrastructure committed to traffic and transportation safety as reparations for the consequences of racism in the housing market a century ago and through the present day.[11] AJPH

CORRESPONDENCE

Correspondence should be sent to Sara F. Jacoby, Department of Family and Community Health, University of Pennsylvania School of Nursing, 418 Curie Boulevard, Philadelphia, PA 19104 (e-mail: sfjacoby@nursing.upenn.edu). Reprints can be ordered at https://ajph.org by clicking the "Reprints" link.

PUBLICATION INFORMATION

Full Citation: Jacoby SF. Home Owners' Loan Corporation maps and place-based injury risks: a complex history. *Am J Public Health*. 2023;113(4): 356–358.

Acceptance Date: January 22, 2023.

DOI: https://doi.org/10.2105/AJPH.2023.307242

CONFLICTS OF INTEREST

The author has no conflicts of interest to disclose.

REFERENCES

1. Baldwin J. The White man's guilt. *Ebony*. August 1965:47.
2. Krieger N. Methods for the scientific study of discrimination and health: an ecosocial approach. *Am J Public Health*. 2012;102(5):936–944. https://doi.org/10.2105/AJPH.2011.300544
3. Hardeman RR, Homan PA, Chantarat T, Davis BA, Brown TH. Improving the measurement of structural racism to achieve antiracist health policy. *Health Aff (Millwood)*. 2022;41(2):179–186. https://doi.org/10.1377/hlthaff.2021.01489
4. Moore M, Conrick KM, Fuentes M, et al. Research on injury disparities: a scoping review. *Health Equity*. 2019;3(1):504–511. https://doi.org/10.1089/heq.2019.0044
5. Nelson RK, Winling L, Marciano R, et al. Mapping Inequality. Eds. Nelson RK, Ayers EL. American Panorama. Available at: https://dsl.richmond.edu/panorama/redlining/#loc=5/39.1/-94.58. Accessed January 2, 2023.
6. Bailey ZD, Krieger N, Agénor M, Graves J, Linos N, Bassett MT. Structural racism and health inequities in the USA: evidence and interventions. *Lancet*. 2017;389(10077):1453–1463. https://doi.org/10.1016/S0140-6736(17)30569-X

7. Gioielli R. The tyranny of the map: rethinking redlining. *The Metropole*. Available at: https://themetropole.blog/2022/11/03/the-tyranny-of-the-map-rethinking-redlining. Accessed January 2, 2023.
8. Hillier AE. Redlining and the Home Owners' Loan Corporation. *J Urban Hist*. 2003;29(4):394–420. https://doi.org/10.1177/0096144203029004002
9. Noelke C, Outrich M, Baek M, et al. Connecting past to present: examining different approaches to linking historical redlining to present day health inequities. *PLoS One*. 2022;17(5):e0267606. https://doi.org/10.1371/journal.pone.0267606
10. Graetz N, Esposito M. Historical redlining and contemporary racial disparities in neighborhood life expectancy. *Soc Forces*. 2022;soac114. https://doi.org/10.1093/sf/soac114
11. Bassett MT, Galea S. Reparations as a public health priority—a strategy for ending Black–White health disparities. *N Engl J Med*. 2020;383(22):2101–2103. https://doi.org/10.1056/NEJMp2026170

Bringing an Equity Lens to Address the Evolving Overdose Crisis: A Public Health of Consequence, April 2023

Farzana Kapadia, PhD, MPH

ABOUT THE AUTHOR

Farzana Kapadia is the deputy editor of AJPH *and professor of epidemiology at the School of Global Public Health, New York University, New York.*

Beginning with the expansion of prescription opioid use in the mid-1990s, the opioid crisis has unfolded in overlapping waves and the United States is now entering its fourth wave of the opioid epidemic (https://bit.ly/3XDslIj). With the evolution of the epidemic, we have witnessed changes in the types of substances driving overdoses and overdose-related deaths, from prescription opioids to heroin and then to synthetic opioids such as fentanyl, to heroin, and now polysubstance use involving both opioids and psychostimulants such as methamphetamines. In this issue of the *Journal*, we present information on trends in methamphetamine-related deaths as well as efforts to reduce overdose-related deaths. These findings highlight the need for ongoing and timely tracking of trends in overdose to ensure an equitable approach to preventing overdose deaths.

METHAMPHETAMINE-RELATED DEATHS

Hoopsick and Yockey (p. 416) provide further evidence on the significant escalation of methamphetamine-related mortality in the United States between 1999 and 2021. In addition to the alarming 58-fold overall increase in methamphetamine-related mortality—from 545 to 32 353 methamphetamine-related deaths between 1999 and 2021—the involvement of heroin with or without fentanyl in these deaths increased by 17.3% annually from 2010 to 2021. These dramatic increases in methamphetamine-related deaths and polysubstance use deaths parallel trends in nonprescription opioid-, synthetic opioid-, and cocaine-related overdose deaths.[1]

DISPARITIES IN OVERDOSE DEATHS

These findings by Hoopsick and Yockey emphasize, once again, the significant burden of overdose deaths in the United States. However, these overall estimates mask disparities in deaths by racial/ethnic background and socioeconomic status indicators, which cannot be ignored. Earlier waves of the opioid epidemic saw increased overdose deaths among younger, White men and women in rural areas. As this crisis continues to evolve, drug use patterns shift; non-Hispanic, Native American Indian and Alaskan Native, and non-Hispanic Black persons now experience higher rates of drug overdose deaths than in prior waves of the opioid epidemic. And although to a lesser degree, overdose deaths have also increased among Hispanic people and Asian/Pacific Islanders in recent waves of the opioid epidemic.

Sociodemographic disparities in overdose and overdose deaths, and the way these disparities have shifted over time, can be traced back to a history of interrelated structural disadvantages that are the fundamental drivers of overdose mortality. These drivers include lower educational attainment, lower income status due to low wages and weak employment opportunities, no or inadequate health insurance coverage, disability status, increasing mental health burdens coupled with inadequate mental health care providers and access to care, and criminal justice involvement.[2] And these factors converged in economically depressed areas across the United States—the Midwest, Appalachia, and the Northeast—creating microepidemics of overdose deaths in states and regions often with already weakened physical and mental health care infrastructure.

The population health impacts of overdose deaths are reverberating across multiple generations. The sharp increase in overdose mortality starting in the 2000s, particularly among adults 25 to 44 years old, has produced a decline in overall life expectancy in the United States since 2014. Deaths due to unintentional injuries, which include overdose-related deaths, have dramatically increased among non-Hispanic

White, non-Hispanic Black, and Hispanic people since 2013.[3] In many cases, grandparents or other available family members are caring for the children of adults who are either unable to care for them or have died from overdose, creating unique economic, social, and health challenges for these caretakers (https://bit.ly/3HfH5Ny) as well as for the children they are raising. Finally, between 2010 and 2017, there has been an 82% increase in infants born with neonatal abstinence syndrome (https://www.cdc.gov/pregnancy/opioids/data.html).

OVERDOSE PREVENTION POLICY

Griffith et al. (p. 372) present findings from an analysis examining the impact of Rhode Island's 2017 statewide mandate that providers prescribe or provide take-home naloxone to anyone presenting to emergency departments (EDs) with opioid overdose. This state mandate, in response to the high rates of overdose mortality in Rhode Island, recognized the need for state-level guidelines to inform delivery of overdose prevention services, to benefit not only patients but also health care organizations and health care systems with uniform guidance and policy on distributing naloxone. Their findings indicate that between 2018 and 2019, 82% of patients presenting to EDs for an overdose were offered naloxone, and that about half of this group accepted a prescription or take-home kit. Receipt of naloxone was associated with a prior ED visit.

From an equity perspective, implementing an "upstream" statewide policy intervention and eliminating naloxone distribution based on provider discretion can achieve greater equity in overdose prevention than "downstream" interventions that focus on individual-level changes. And although the study results indicate no major differences in naloxone uptake across demographic groups, an ED intervention by its nature means that it is only available for those patients who are able to access an ED. Rather than considering this an inadequate policy intervention, it may be viewed as one of many necessary policy interventions that seek to undo the harms wrought by legacies of institutional advantages and disadvantages that affect population-level health.

Moreover, changes in drug supply and drug demand have shaped, and will continue to shape, the evolution of overdose and overdose deaths in the United States, and require harm reduction approaches to adapt quickly and appropriately. Most recently, a *New York Times* article (https://nyti.ms/3wbpobN) reported that increased use of xylazine, a sedative used by veterinarians, along with fentanyl is increasing health risks to persons who use drugs, and is challenging current harm reduction efforts.

A HEALTH EQUITY RESPONSE TO THE OVERDOSE CRISIS

As the overdose crisis in the United States continues to evolve, with new and more potent substances introduced into the US drug supply, we need to double down on our commitment to providing a comprehensive and health equity–motivated public health approach to address this crisis.[4] The first step begins with redoubling our efforts to reduce the stigma and discrimination experienced by persons who use drugs to prevent exacerbating inequalities. Next, decriminalizing possession of drugs and criminal justice reform are two necessary policy actions that can reduce racial and ethnic disparities in the overdose crisis. Finally, expansion of prevention and treatment efforts that are community based and that respect and rely on the knowledge of persons who use drugs will have greater impact on reducing health inequalities and drug overdose. AJPH

CORRESPONDENCE

Correspondence should be sent to Farzana Kapadia, PhD, MPH, New York University, School of Global Public Health, 708 Broadway, Room 729, New York, NY 10003 (e-mail: farzana.kapadia@nyu.edu). Reprints can be ordered at http://www.ajph.org by clicking the "Reprints" link.

PUBLICATION INFORMATION

Full Citation: Kapadia F. Bringing an equity lens to address the evolving overdose crisis: a public health of consequence, April 2023. *Am J Public Health*. 2023;113(4):359–360.

Acceptance Date: January 21, 2023.

DOI: https://doi.org/10.2105/AJPH.2023.307240

CONFLICTS OF INTEREST

The author has no conflicts of interest to disclose.

REFERENCES

1. Spencer MR, Miniño AM, Warner M. *Drug Overdose Deaths in the United States, 2001–2021*. Hyattsville, MD: National Center for Health Statistics; 2022. NCHS Data Brief no. 457. https://doi.org/10.15620/cdc:122556
2. Dasgupta N, Beletsky L, Ciccarone D. Opioid crisis: no easy fix to its social and economic determinants. *Am J Public Health*. 2018;108(2):182–186. https://doi.org/10.2105/AJPH.2017.304187
3. Curtin SC, Xu JQ. *Death Rates for Leading Causes of Death for People Aged 25–44 Among the Three Largest Race and Ethnicity Groups: United States, 2000–2020*. Hyattsville, MD: National Center for Health Statistics; 2022. NCHS Data Brief no. 451. https://doi.org/10.15620/cdc:121796
4. Hansen H, Netherland J. Is the prescription opioid epidemic a white problem? *Am J Public Health*. 2016;106(12):2127–2129. https://doi.org/10.2105/AJPH.2016.303483

Improving the US and Global Pandemic Response: Lessons From Cuba

Sandro Galea, MD, DrPH, and Paul C. Erwin, MD, DrPH

ABOUT THE AUTHORS

Sandro Galea is with the School of Public Health, Boston University, Boston, MA. Paul C. Erwin is with the School of Public Health, University of Alabama at Birmingham and is an associate editor of AJPH.

At this point, it is abundantly clear that the global response to the COVID-19 pandemic has fallen far short of what we might have hoped. More than six million people have died globally from COVID-19, with more than a million of those deaths in the United States. The United States has had more deaths by far than any other country worldwide. Although there probably is no one country that can claim to have performed well in all dimensions of its COVID-19 response, there are some countries that did better than others on important dimensions of the response, and it behooves us to start the process of learning from these countries toward the end of improving both US and global responses in the inevitable event of future pandemics.

Such lessons can be drawn from the recently published report "Cuba's COVID-19 Vaccine Enterprise: Report From a High-Level Fact-Finding Delegation to Cuba."[1] This international delegation was organized by Medical Education Cooperation with Cuba (MEDICC), a US-based nonprofit that promotes health-related dialogue and collaboration, especially between the United States and Cuba.[2] Cuba had substantially lower mortality during the COVID-19 pandemic, with about 750 deaths per million, comparable with New Zealand, a country that has often been spotlighted for its handling of the pandemic. The report is an efficient summary of Cuba's success in two particular dimensions during COVID-19 that contributed to its weathering the pandemic as well as it did: Cuba's ability to develop an effective vaccine rapidly, and its ability to subsequently vaccinate a large portion (> 90%) of its population quickly. Although we leave it to the reader to read the MEDICC report, we suggest that there are three key observations that emerge from the report that are helpful to bear in mind as we consider how to improve the US national pandemic response.

First, much of the success of vaccine development and vaccine delivery built on decades of investment in both areas. Rapid vaccine development was possible because Cuba has been investing in its biotech sector for 40 years. This has had previous successes (e.g., vaccines against Haemophilus influenzae type b and serogroup B meningococcus) on which the country was able to build its COVID-19 vaccine development. This history of prior investment in biomedical technology is not substantially different from such investment in the United States, and both rapidly yielded effective vaccines. However, Cuba has also invested in a primary care system that provides the infrastructure for delivery of health care on which vaccination efforts were built. We have long known that access to a primary care provider is one of the central determinants of vaccination; that access, long built into the Cuban health care system, has become invaluable for the delivery of vaccines. Moreover, Cuba's primary care system served as the vehicle for its COVID vaccine clinical trials, allowing for countrywide implementation, with results immediately available to the *Ministerio de Salud Pública* (Ministry of Public Health) for subsequent scaling up and widescale deployment.[3]

Second, Cuba's successes were dependent on national central investment and coordination both of vaccine development and delivery efforts. This is in stark contrast with US efforts, which were characterized by deeply fragmented systems, particularly when it came to vaccine delivery. Cuba here clearly has the advantage of being a much smaller country than the United States. However, US states that are smaller than Cuba suffered from fragmentation of service delivery, showing that size was not the only factor leading to the failure of the US COVID-19 response. Rather, a lesson from the Cuban experience is that it is difficult to deal with an epidemic without a national coordinated response that applies standards across the country in a manner that is data-driven and evidence-informed. Cuba was able to do that in part through a history of building a centralized health care infrastructure that provided the pillars on which a nationally coordinated response could be built. That should offer much encouragement for a careful consideration of comparable centralized efforts to deal with future epidemic responses in the United States. In retrospect, one of the shortcomings of the initial US COVID-19 vaccine delivery was the failure to include primary health care providers; because of the trust people have in them, their involvement from the outset might have prevented much of the subsequent vaccine hesitancy we have experienced.

Third, the ongoing economic and social isolation of Cuba because of US-imposed restrictions hindered both Cuba's and the world's efforts to respond to the COVID-19 pandemic. Cuba was developing approaches, including vaccines, that could have helped global efforts to vaccinate as large a proportion of the world's population as possible, as quickly as possible. These efforts were available principally to countries with preexisting ties to Cuba and offered little help to the broader global community. Because US restrictions on Cuba extend to other countries, those without preexisting ties to Cuba could not benefit from either the Cuban vaccines or boosters. Similarly, the isolation of the Cuban scientific community resulted in fewer articles published documenting the successes in Cuba, therefore limiting the lessons learned and the generalizability of the Cuban experience. Conversely, as has often been the case because of its economic isolation, Cuba was inventing approaches to dealing with COVID-19 out of whole cloth, not benefiting much from approaches—including vaccine technology—that were gaining rapid prominence in the United States and other countries. In the context of a pandemic that does not respect artificial human-made borders, the persistence of human-made limits on commerce and knowledge hampers our ability as a global community to adopt the best possible strategies, incurring loss to human life in the process.

It is always important when discussing medical and public health successes to ask, at what cost was success achieved? This is particularly the case in a country like Cuba, whose communist political system has been opposed by the United States for more than 60 years. And yet, the development of effective vaccine and vaccination efforts has little to do with political systems and should not diminish our interest in learning from Cuban approaches, or our commitment to helping Cuba build a healthier country, grounded in human rights. One might hope that a global pandemic can be the catalyst for transcending both borders and long entrenched political perspectives that can hold back health both in Cuba and in the United States. AJPH

CORRESPONDENCE

Correspondence should be sent to Paul C. Erwin, MD, DrPH, Dean and Professor, School of Public Health, the University of Alabama at Birmingham, 1665 University Blvd, RPHB 140B, Birmingham, AL 35294-0022 (e-mail: perwin@uab.edu). Reprints can be ordered at http://www.ajph.org by clicking the "Reprints" link.

PUBLICATION INFORMATION

Full Citation: Galea S, Erwin PC. Improving the US and global pandemic response: lessons from Cuba. *Am J Public Health*. 2023;113(4):361–362.

Acceptance Date: January 9, 2023.

DOI: https://doi.org/10.2105/AJPH.2023.307229

CONTRIBUTORS

S. Galea completed an initial draft. Both authors participated fully in subsequent writing, editing, and revising, and approved the final version.

CONFLICTS OF INTEREST

Paul C. Erwin is a board member of the Medical Education Cooperation With Cuba (MEDICC) but was not involved in the work of the delegation as described in this editorial.

REFERENCES

1. Medical Education Cooperation With Cuba. Cuba's COVID-19 vaccine enterprise: report from a high-level fact-finding delegation to Cuba. 2022. Available at: http://mediccreview.org/executive-summary-insights-from-cubas-covid-19-vaccine-enterprise. Accessed January 4, 2023.
2. Medical Education Cooperation With Cuba. Available at: http://medicc.org/ns. Accessed January 4, 2023.
3. Reed G. Putting science to work: Cuba's COVID-19 pandemic experience. 2022. Available at: http://mediccreview.org/wp-content/uploads/2022/10/MR2022-Vol24-N3%E2%80%934.pdf. Accessed January 4, 2023.

Identifying COVID-19 Vaccine Deserts and Ways to Reduce Them: A Digital Tool to Support Public Health Decision-Making

Rebecca L. Weintraub, MD, Kate Miller, PhD, MPH, Benjamin Rader, MPH, Julie Rosenberg, MPH, Shreyas Srinath, MS, Samuel R. Woodbury, BA, Marinanicole D. Schultheiss, MPH, Mansi Kansal, MBA, Swapnil Vispute, MS, Stylianos Serghiou, MD, PhD, Gerardo Flores, BA, Akim Kumok, MS, Tomer Shekel, MBA, Evgeniy Gabrilovich, PhD, Iman Ahmad, BS, Molly E. Chiang, and John S. Brownstein, PhD

A private–academic partnership built the Vaccine Equity Planner (VEP) to help decision-makers improve geographic access to COVID-19 vaccinations across the United States by identifying vaccine deserts and facilities that could fill those deserts. The VEP presented complex, updated data in an intuitive form during a rapidly changing pandemic situation. The persistence of vaccine deserts in every state as COVID-19 booster recommendations develop suggests that vaccine delivery can be improved. Underresourced public health systems benefit from tools providing real-time, accurate, actionable data. (*Am J Public Health*. 2023; 113(4):363–367. https://doi.org/10.2105/AJPH.2022.307198)

AJPH April 2023, Vol 113, No. 4

Public health leaders can make better, more equitable decisions when they can clearly see and understand the problems. Being presented with potential solutions based on evidence further supports their decision-making and can aid in supporting health equity.

INTERVENTION AND IMPLEMENTATION

We built the Vaccine Equity Planner (VEP) in spring 2021. We intended the VEP to serve US public health planners as an open-access online tool with four main functions:

1. Identify COVID-19 vaccine deserts for both adults and children;
2. Identify facilities within vaccine deserts that could serve as vaccination sites;
3. Focus on specific geographic areas, such as those with high social vulnerability; and
4. Estimate the size of the unvaccinated population in each county as well as the population's intention to be vaccinated.

We plotted all active COVID-19 vaccination site locations, calculating a catchment area around each site based on the amount of time to reach that site by different methods of transportation (walking, public transit, driving). We defined "vaccine deserts" as areas that did not fall within the catchment area of any in-state vaccination site.[1] To identify potential vaccination sites in the deserts, we used publicly available, national, updated data sets of facilities that people would "very likely" trust to get vaccinated: doctors' offices, pharmacies, community health clinics, schools, grocery stores, and churches or religious centers. We repeated this process using only vaccination sites offering the Pfizer age 12 years and up vaccine and the Pfizer age 5–11 years vaccine (the only vaccines available under emergency use authorization for the pediatric population at the time) to create pediatric vaccine deserts. As vaccines were approved for different age demographics, we added additional displays to the tool.

We overlaid our map with data from the Social Vulnerability Index and data on intention to be vaccinated from the COVID-19 Trends and Impact Survey (for full data sources and methods, see Appendix A, available as a supplement to the online version of this article at http://www.ajph.org). We sought feedback from potential users and refined the design and tool accordingly.

We directly disseminated the VEP by e-mail to all state- and jurisdiction-level health commissioners with publicly available contact information and shared the tool on social media. Several leaders and the Association of Immunization Managers responded to our communications with requests for training on the tool, specific data, updates to the tool, or other queries, which we addressed.

PLACE, TIME, AND PERSONS

Our target user was a state or county public health planner in the United States who wanted to expand geographic access to COVID-19 vaccination in their jurisdiction. We refreshed data on vaccination sites, vaccine deserts, and potential vaccination sites weekly starting in June 2021 as demand for vaccination fell.

PURPOSE

Vaccines reduce hospitalization and the risk of escape variants, supporting pandemic response.[2] The World Health Organization (WHO) has classified vaccine hesitancy into "three Cs": people may lack confidence in the effectiveness or safety of the vaccine, may feel complacent about the risk and severity of the disease, or may not have convenient access to the vaccine.[3] In the United States, these three Cs vary, resulting in inequitable uptake of vaccines and, in turn, differential disease burden of COVID-19.[4]

One common method for understanding convenience or geographic access to services is the "desert," an area devoid of the service in question. Unfortunately, in spring 2021, few US public health departments had the bandwidth available to collect and analyze data from disparate sources to identify COVID-19 deserts and potential ways to ameliorate them.

To provide planners with the necessary data for increasing equitable access to COVID-19 vaccines, members from Ariadne Labs, the Computational Epidemiology Lab at Boston Children's

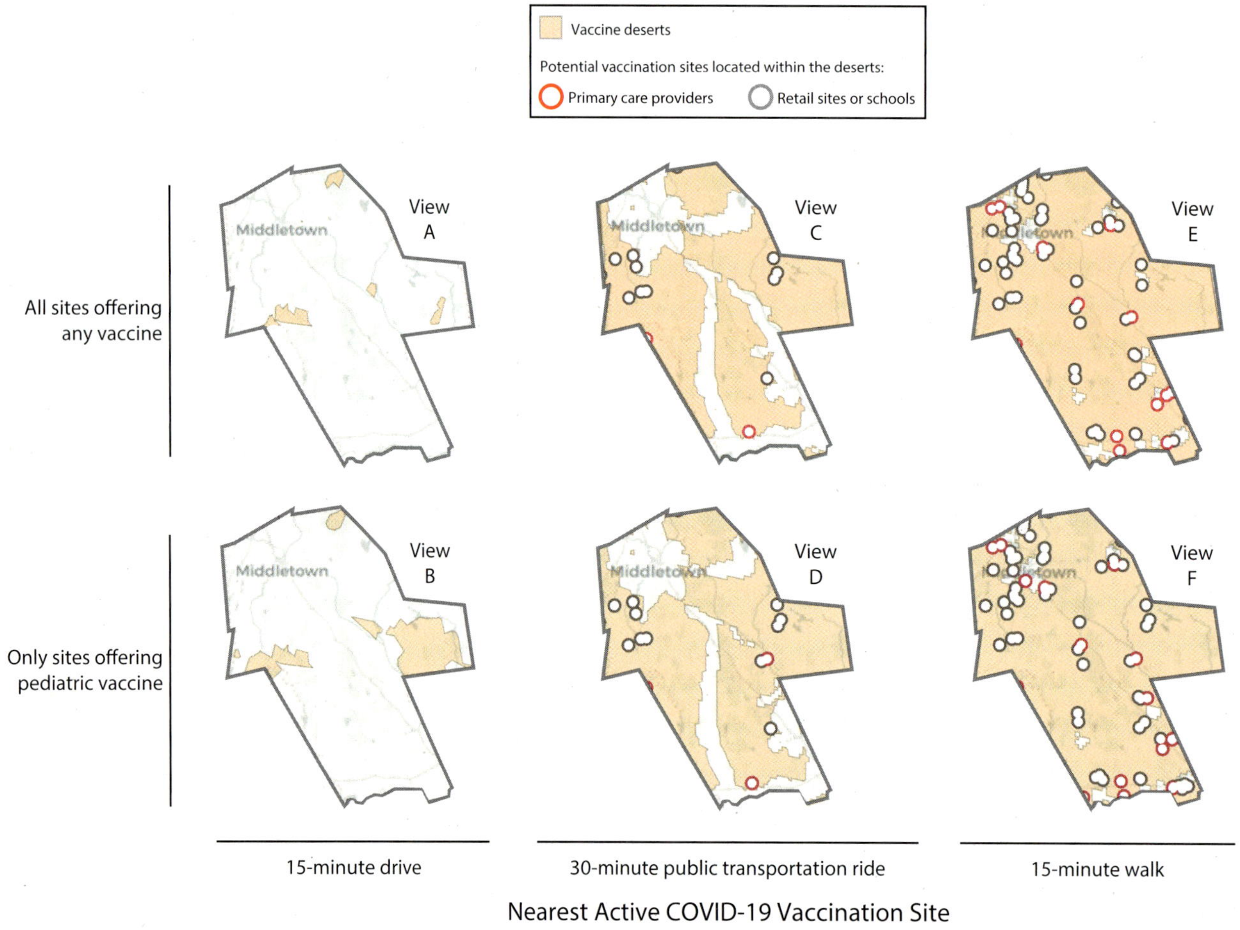

FIGURE 1— Vaccine Deserts in 1 Sample US County, by Travel Mode, Travel Time, and Vaccine Type: November 10, 2022

Note. A vaccine desert is an area that does not have access to an active COVID-19 site within the time and by the transportation method selected.

Hospital, and Google collaborated to gather, curate, and display data from various public sources. The aim was to identify COVID-19 deserts and potential vaccination sites within those deserts as well as share the population's social vulnerability and intentions to be vaccinated. The goal was to enable better-informed public health planning and decision-making.

EVALUATION AND ADVERSE EFFECTS

We launched the VEP on May 24, 2021. By September 20, 2021, it had roughly 7400 unique page views originating within the United States. Nearly 70% of the incoming Web traffic originated from direct entry of the URL to a browser, suggesting that spread occurred through our communication campaign and word of mouth.

Vaccine Deserts

Vaccine deserts existed in every US state, but the extent and location of those deserts depended on the chosen transportation mode and travel time. In general, vaccine deserts were more expansive when the transportation mode was public transit or walking. Additionally, pediatric vaccine deserts tended to be more expansive than adult vaccine deserts because not all vaccination sites offered the Pfizer age 5–11 years vaccine. Many vaccine deserts had one or more potential vaccination sites, including primary care sites, schools, and retail sites (Figure 1, county anonymized).

Potential Vaccination Sites Located in Deserts

Over 13 weeks with available data, the VEP identified approximately 21 000 potential vaccination sites across the United States. Most of these sites were places of worship (10 000), schools (7000–8000), or retail sites (1000). The smallest categories—with fewer than 1000 potential sites each—included health-related facilities that were not already providing COVID-19 vaccination: primary care sites, federally qualified health centers, and pharmacies (Figure 2).

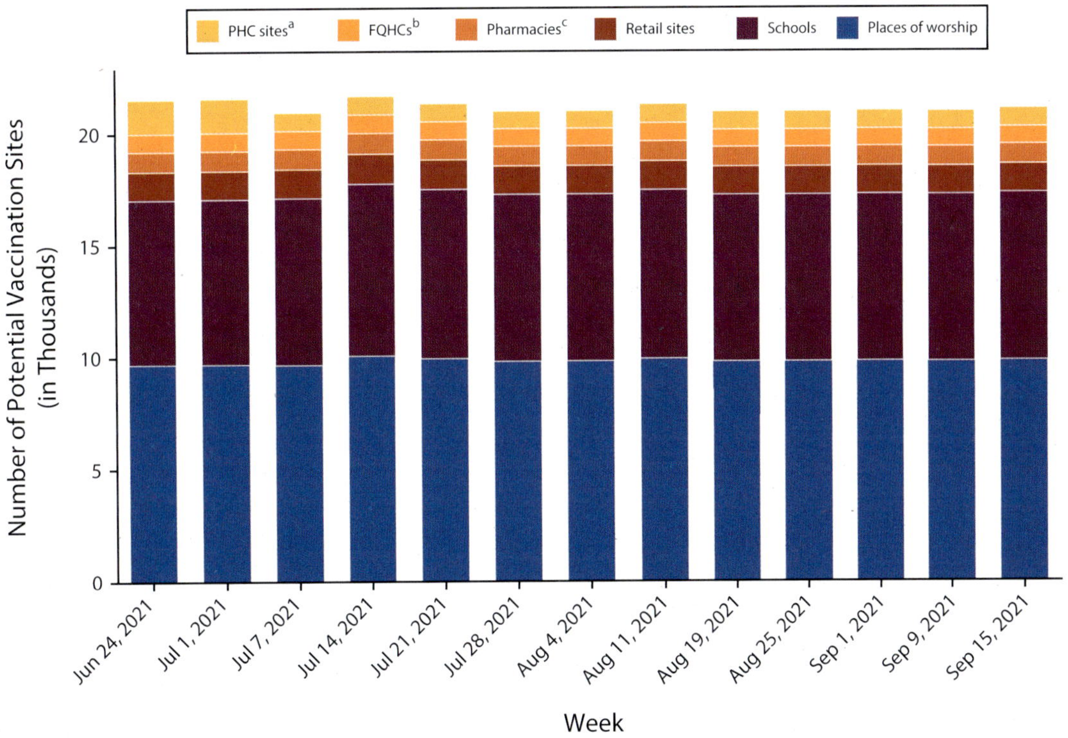

FIGURE 2— Number of Potential Vaccination Sites Located in Vaccine Deserts, by Week and Type of Site: United States, June 24–September 15, 2021

Note. FQHC = Federally qualified health center; PHC = Primary health care. A vaccine desert is an area outside a 15-minute drive to the nearest active COVID-19 vaccination site.

[a]Includes family medicine physicians, internal medicine physicians, pediatricians, and general practitioners.
[b]FQHC not already vaccinating.
[c]Pharmacies not already vaccinating.

SUSTAINABILITY

There is great potential for intersectoral partnerships to support public health leaders by leveraging data, analytic, communication, and technological skills to generate evidence to support decision-making. The VEP continues to support the Association of Immunization Managers in increasing vaccine access across its jurisdictions.

PUBLIC HEALTH SIGNIFICANCE

The VEP revealed vaccine deserts in every US state. In general, it showed that vaccine deserts were more common in rural areas, and many potential vaccination sites within these deserts were schools; however, there are also many untapped medical clinics.

A successful response to the COVID-19 pandemic is supported by widespread, equitable access to the COVID-19 vaccines. Geographic access is necessary to the WHO's convenience factor and is a potentially powerful lever for increasing equity of access. Surveys have found that 15% of unvaccinated people are concerned about the difficulty of traveling to a vaccination site, and 20% are concerned about the need to take time off work, which would be exacerbated by long travel times.[4] Additionally, geographic access can support the confidence of unvaccinated people: 53% of unvaccinated people report that they were more likely to accept the vaccine from their own trusted health care provider, such as a primary health care site, family medicine physician, or pediatrician, compared with other types of sites.[5] Improving local access leads to local reporting from friends and neighbors communicating why they got vaccinated and boosted, and the unvaccinated are influenced by their peers.[6]

In the rapid deployment of COVID-19 vaccines in the United States, the barriers to equitable distribution were numerous and closely related to larger structural barriers in public health delivery.[7] Planners had to consider a population's confidence and complacency regarding vaccines, as well as to promote convenient access, which would support equitable distribution to the most vulnerable.[3,8] Meeting these goals required a certain bandwidth to analyze data, understand needs, and plan accordingly. After months of battling the pandemic, not all public health departments in the United States had the time or resources to do so. For our part, we will consider applying what we have learned from building the VEP to display other clinical and service deserts. The VEP was built through a partnership between academia and the private sector, and further investment is needed to promote such collaboration to build tools to support data-driven public health decision-making. AJPH

ABOUT THE AUTHORS

At the time of this work, Rebecca L. Weintraub, Kate Miller, Julie Rosenberg, Shreyas Srinath, Samuel R. Woodbury, and Iman Ahmad were with Ariadne Labs, Boston, MA. Benjamin Rader, Marinanicole D. Schultheiss, Molly E. Chiang, and John S. Brownstein were with Computational Epidemiology Lab, Boston Children's Hospital, Boston. Mansi Kansal, Swapnil Vispute, Stylianos Serghiou, Gerardo Flores, Akim Kumok, Tomer Shekel, and Evgeniy Gabrilovich were with Google Inc, Mountain View, CA.

CORRESPONDENCE

Correspondence should be sent to Rebecca L. Weintraub, 401 Park Dr, 3rd Fl, Boston, MA 02215 (e-mail: rlweintraub@bwh.harvard.edu). Reprints can be ordered at http://www.ajph.org by clicking the "Reprints" link.

PUBLICATION INFORMATION

Full Citation: Weintraub RL, Miller K, Rader B, et al. Identifying COVID-19 vaccine deserts and ways to reduce them: a digital tool to support public health decision-making. *Am J Public Health*. 2023;113(4):363–367.

Acceptance Date: December 3, 2022.

DOI: https://doi.org/10.2105/AJPH.2022.307198

CONTRIBUTORS

Study conceptualization and methodology activities were conducted by R. L. Weintraub, K. Miller, B. Rader, J. Rosenberg, M. Schultheiss, M. Kansal, S. Vispute, S. Serghiou, T. Shekel, E. Gabrilovich, I. Ahmad, M. E. Chiang, and J. S. Brownstein. Data curation, formal analysis, investigation, provision of resources, and software activities were conducted by R. L. Weintraub, K. Miller, B. Rader, J. Rosenberg, S. Srinath, S. Woodbury, M. Kansal, S. Vispute, S. Serghiou, G. Flores, A. Kumok, I. Ahmad, M. E. Chiang, and J. S. Brownstein. Funding acquisition and supervision activities were conducted by R. L. Weintraub, K. Miller, B. Rader, J. Rosenberg, M. Kansal, E. Gabrilovich, and J. S. Brownstein. Visualization activities were conducted by R. L. Weintraub, K. Miller, J. Rosenberg, S. Srinath, S. Woodbury, and S. Vispute. Project administration activities were conducted by R. L. Weintraub, J. Rosenberg, M. Schultheiss, M. Kansal, T. Shekel, and I. Ahmad. R. L. Weintraub, B. Rader, J. Rosenberg, M. Schultheiss, and E. Gabrilovich wrote the original draft. All authors reviewed and approved the final draft.

ACKNOWLEDGMENTS

The Ariadne Labs COVID-19 Vaccine Delivery team was funded in part by The Commonwealth Fund. The Computational Epidemiology Lab at Boston Children's Hospital was funded in part by the Centers for Disease Control and Prevention, Facebook, and The Rockefeller Foundation. HealthLandscape provided some of the data used.

Thank you to all reviewers and public health leaders who provided feedback.

CONFLICTS OF INTEREST

The authors have no conflicts of interest to disclose.

HUMAN PARTICIPANT PROTECTION

No human participants were involved in the conduct of this research. Therefore, this study has not been subject to review by an institutional review board.

REFERENCES

1. Rader B, Astley CM, Sewalk K, et al. Spatial accessibility modeling of vaccine deserts as barriers to controlling SARS-CoV-2. *medRxiv*. Published online June 12, 2021. https://doi.org/10.1101/2021.06.09.21252858
2. Read AF, Baigent SJ, Powers C, et al. Imperfect vaccination can enhance the transmission of highly virulent pathogens. *PLoS Biol*. 2015;13(7):e1002198. https://doi.org/10.1371/journal.pbio.1002198
3. SAGE Working Group. *Report of the SAGE Working Group on Vaccine Hesitancy*. Geneva, Switzerland: World Health Organization; 2014.

4. Kaiser Family Foundation. Latest data on COVID-19 vaccinations by race/ethnicity. Available at: https://www.kff.org/coronavirus-covid-19/issue-brief/latest-data-on-covid-19-vaccinations-race-ethnicity. Accessed September 23, 2021.
5. American COVID-19 Vaccine Poll. Available at: https://covidvaccinepoll.com/app/aarc/covid-19-vaccine-messaging/#. Accessed October 8, 2021.
6. Schneider KE, Dayton L, Rouhani S, Latkin CA. Implications of attitudes and beliefs about COVID-19 vaccines for vaccination campaigns in the United States: a latent class analysis. *Prev Med Rep.* 2021;24:101584. https://doi.org/10.1016/j.pmedr.2021.101584
7. Shen AK, Hughes Iv R, DeWald E, Rosenbaum S, Pisani A, Orenstein W. Ensuring equitable access to COVID-19 vaccines in the US: current system challenges and opportunities. *Health Aff (Millwood).* 2021;40(1):62–69. https://doi.org/10.1377/hlthaff.2020.01554
8. Kaiser Family Foundation. KFF COVID-19 vaccine monitor: experiences with vaccine access and information needs. Available at: https://www.kff.org/coronavirus-covid-19/poll-finding/kff-covid-19-vaccine-monitor-experiences-vaccine-access-information-needs. Accessed October 8, 2021.

Improving Early Childhood Caries for American Indian 3- to 5-Year-Old Children Through Interprofessional Outreach: 2018–2022

Laura S. Larsson, RN, PhD, MPH, and Christine Hodgson, RN, PhD, MSN, CPNP-PC

We sought to determine the effectiveness of an interprofessional health team in improving access to oral health care among American Indian children enrolled in Head Start. Our team provided preventive treatments and case management during 11 visits from 2018 to 2022. Case management reduced the time between referral and dental treatment from a median of 166 days to 58.3 days over four years. An interprofessional team is an effective way to improve access to oral health care among rural American Indian Head Start children. (*Am J Public Health*. 2023;113(4):368–371. https://doi.org/10.2105/AJPH.2022.307205)

AJPH April 2023, Vol 113, No. 4

Dental and public health experts have drawn attention to the persistent disparities with respect to early childhood caries (ECC) among American Indian and Alaska Native (AI/AN) children over the past 20 years and called for better prevention efforts and an interdisciplinary approach. Current recommendations emphasize increased integration of oral health education and preventive care in early childhood intervention programming.

INTERVENTION AND IMPLEMENTATION

Our interprofessional team delivered an intervention over four years with a Tribal Head Start program to address gaps in access to dental care among young children. The goals were to reduce rates of untreated decay and to decrease the time to dental treatment. Services included prophylaxis, fluoride varnish application, dental sealant placement and repair, and silver diamine fluoride application. Also, in response to COVID-19, we added synchronous and asynchronous teledentistry in November 2020 including X-rays, intraoral photos, limited examinations, and consultations.

Our team consisted of nursing students, nurse practitioners, a project coordinator, and dental hygienists who traveled to eight Head Start classrooms in the fall, winter, and spring. All children were assessed for vision and hearing acuity, oral health status, height, and weight. We employed case management principles including oral health guidance to families and assistance in making appointments.

At each visit, we provided a letter to parents and oral health supplies for home and supervised twice-daily classroom brushing. Services were free of charge to families; however, Montana Medicaid was billed for those with public insurance.

PLACE, TIME, AND PERSONS

The goals of Tribal Head Start are to offer preschool nutrition services and family support services for low-income children three to five years of age who live on Native American lands. Children in the study (n = 475) attended the Northern Cheyenne Tribal Head Start program between 2018 and 2022. The Northern Cheyenne Nation, home to 5000 Montana residents, includes parts of Rosebud and Big Horn counties, both designated as dental professional shortage areas.[1]

PURPOSE

ECC (commonly known as tooth decay), the most prevalent infectious disease among children, is rooted in both individual and environmental factors.[2] The prevalence of ECC is high among preschool-aged children across the United States but as much as five times higher among AI/AN preschoolers than among preschoolers in general.[3,4] In addition, AI/AN children have decay that presents earlier and is more severe.[3]

Although the epidemiology of ECC among indigenous children is complex, access to care is the most glaring obstacle to oral health in Montana's AI communities. Eleven of Montana's 56 counties lack a residing dentist, and 86 locations are designated dental shortage areas.[1] In response, the American Academy of Pediatrics[3] and the State of Montana Oral Health Strategic Plan[5] have recommended integration of oral health education, preventive care, and an interdisciplinary approach involving the Special Supplemental Nutrition Program for Women, Infants, and Children; Head Start; and other maternal and child programs.[6] Further recommendations include workforce expansion[7,8] and having allied health care providers operate to their full scope of practice.[9,10]

EVALUATION AND ADVERSE EFFECTS

Our team visited classrooms during the fall, winter, and spring of each year except during 2020–2021, when we visited only twice because of the pandemic. We provided 313 cleanings, 442 fluoride varnish applications, 801 sealant placements or repairs, and 99 applications of silver diamine fluoride for 475 preschoolers. We referred 161 children, of whom 123 completed treatment (76.4%; 59 boys).

The median number of days between referral and treatment improved over the project period from 166 days to 58.3 days (Figure 1 and Table A, available as a supplement to the online version of this article at http://www.ajph.org). Outdated telephone numbers, long distances to dentists, and disappointment when the first appointment is a consultation rather than treatment are ongoing challenges to prompt treatment.

ECC rates (mean = 58.7%; SD = 4.0%) remained stable over the project period relative to the baseline rate of 57.4% and remained below the 71.3% national average among AI/AN children three to five years old. This rate was above the 24.9% rate among White children.[4] The average untreated caries rate was 33.8% (SD = 10.7%), which was below the 37.7% baseline rate, below the 43.4% national average among AI/AN children three to five years of age, and higher than the 10.0% rate among White children.[4] Untreated caries rates stayed below the national benchmark for the first eight visits but exceeded the national average for the final three visits (with rates of 62.9%, 53.6%, and 46.7%), when supervised classroom toothbrushing was suspended during the COVID-19 pandemic (Figure 2). The associated increase in caries rates is noteworthy. New guidance for reopened classroom toothbrushing emphasizes safety for children and staff with children brushing at their desks rather than at the sink.[11] This not only reduces transmission of droplets but increases the time fluoride is on the teeth.

The program offered benefits for students as well as the Head Start

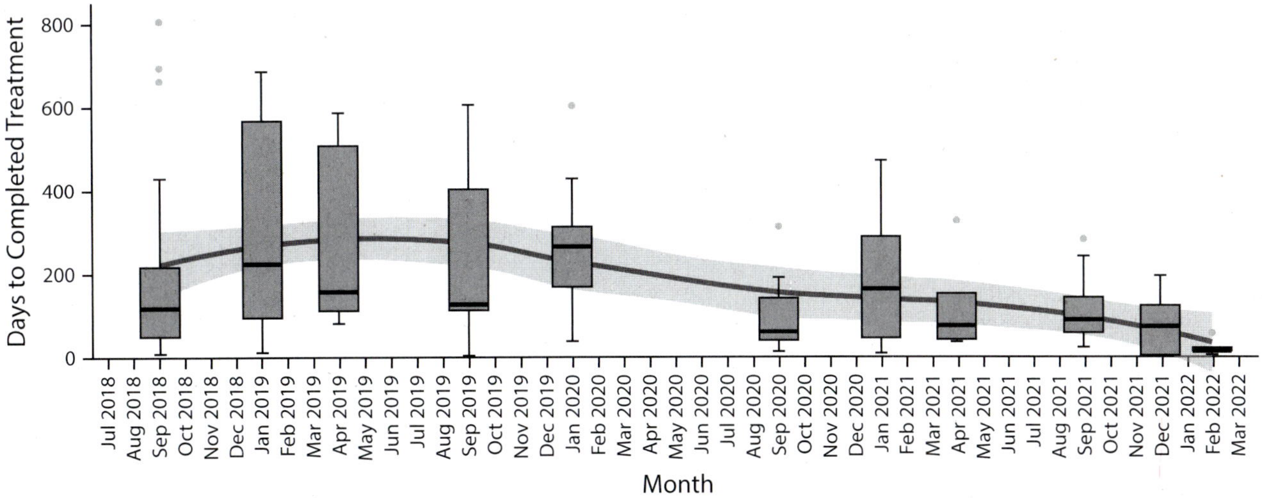

FIGURE 1— Variations in Time to Treatment Among Northern Cheyenne Nation Head Start Children Referred to Dental Treatment: Montana, 2018–2022

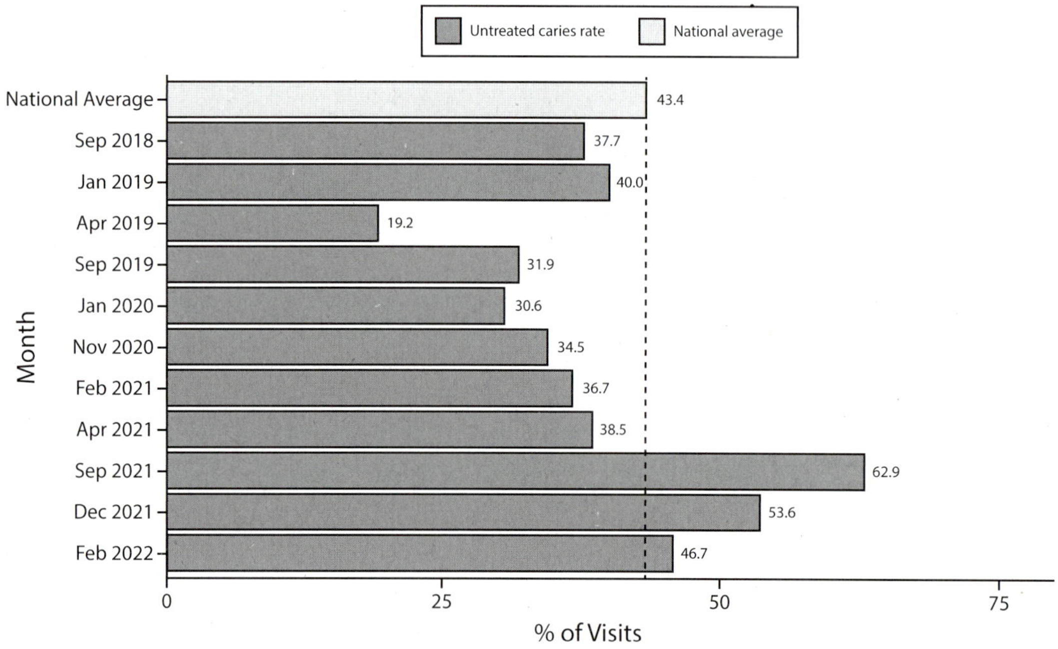

FIGURE 2— Untreated Caries Rates Among Northern Cheyenne Nation Head Start Children, by Visit, Relative to the 2019 National Average: Montana, 2018–2022

Note. In April 2019, the classroom caries rate was 19.2%, which was 24.2 percentage points less than the national benchmark.[4]

program. At the outset of the project, the Head Start program was challenged to meet health program performance standards. Today, the program is in compliance with completion rates for medical examinations (74%), hearing examinations (79%), vision screenings (81%), and dental screenings (82%).[12]

SUSTAINABILITY

Our integrated team of nursing students, nurse practitioners, dental hygienists, and tribal leaders was able to establish a sustainable model that is expanding to three other AI communities in the new project period (2022–2026). Our team will grow to include an educational therapist and a psychiatric mental health nurse practitioner to help Head Start comply with required developmental assessments and interventions.

The Northern Cheyenne Nation invited us to provide school-based care in its kindergarten through 12th-grade classrooms, where wrap-around services can be enhanced with monthly clinics. These expansions are funded through a combination of federal, state, and private grants, but we see this as a transitional measure. The tribal health department is currently activating an agreement in which it will contract with the Indian Health Service to independently provide health care services using the provisions of the Indian Self Determination Act. With planning for this transition under way, the department will be able to conduct third-party billing for these school-based services while contracting with the nurse-led interprofessional team to provide care.

PUBLIC HEALTH SIGNIFICANCE

Two lessons from this study suggest that community-based research can result in immediate action, far earlier than upon dissemination of results. First, one sociopolitical effect of this study occurred when the state of Montana expanded the authorization to apply silver diamine fluoride to limited-access permit-endorsed dental hygienists operating under general supervision of the team dentist. Our inaugural application of silver diamine fluoride was in September 2019, and the results demonstrate that enhancing the autonomy of dental hygienists is both safe and effective. Second, because of the COVID-19 pandemic, we successfully implemented the use of teledentistry to address gaps in access to care among AI children enrolled in a Head Start program in a rural area.

The results from our study support the hypothesis that receipt of care from the interprofessional team would have reduced Head Start preschool children's time to treatment by a dentist after identification of ECC. Reduced time to treatment is significant in that it reflects reduced pain from dental caries along with other effects of ECC on young children such as eating disturbances, speech and language issues, school attendance, and missed work for parents.

Our study demonstrated the success of an interprofessional team in providing critical dental services. The partnership among tribal communities, university researchers, and clinicians has served as a model for this program to grow across the state of Montana. Since initiation of the intervention, we have reached four tribal nations and prepared five campuses of nursing students for rural practice. We have developed a curriculum addressing social determinants of health, medical–dental integration, and multicultural care. In the literature,[3,6,10] effectiveness of mobile dental units partnering with schools and Head Start programs has a convincing evidence base. Our results suggest that interprofessional teams with members operating to their full scope of practice not only provide missing pieces to the puzzle of access to dental care in rural areas but bring oral health into the whole picture of school readiness, overall health, and general well-being. AJPH

ABOUT THE AUTHORS

Laura S. Larsson is with the Mark & Robyn Jones College of Nursing, Montana State University, Bozeman. Christine Hodgson is with the College of Nursing, University of Arizona, Tucson.

CORRESPONDENCE

Correspondence should be sent to Laura S. Larsson, 173560 APS Hall, Bozeman, MT 59717 (e-mail: llarsson@montana.edu). Reprints can be ordered at http://www.ajph.org by clicking the "Reprints" link.

PUBLICATION INFORMATION

Full Citation: Larsson LS, Hodgson C. Improving early childhood caries for American Indian 3- to 5-year-old children through interprofessional outreach: 2018–2022. *Am J Public Health*. 2023; 113(4):368–371.

Acceptance Date: December 12, 2022.

DOI: https://doi.org/10.2105/AJPH.2022.307205

CONTRIBUTORS

L. S. Larsson originated the study, collected and analyzed the data, wrote the results section, and revised and edited drafts of the article. C. Hodgson wrote the review of literature, methods, and implications sections and revised and edited drafts of the article.

ACKNOWLEDGMENTS

We acknowledge Crystal Spring and the Smiles Across Montana team; Emily Killsback, Roberta Harris, and Lanita LittleWhiteman at Northern Cheyenne Head Start; Mina Seminole, tribal liaison to the project; and the following funders who were all essential to this work: Montana Innovations in Prevention (grant HRSA-18-014); the Nurse Education, Practice, Quality and Retention Program (grant HRSA UK1HP31719); the Otto Bremer Trust; Blue Cross Blue Shield Healthy Kids Healthy Families; the Dennis & Phyllis Washington Foundation; and AstraZeneca.

CONFLICTS OF INTEREST

The authors have no potential or actual conflicts of interest to disclose.

HUMAN PARTICIPANT PROTECTION

Informed consent documents and the research process were approved by Chief Dull Knife College and Montana State University.

REFERENCES

1. Health Resources and Services Administration. Shortage areas. Available at: https://data.hrsa.gov/topics/health-workforce/shortage-areas. Accessed September 22, 2022.
2. National Institute of Dental and Craniofacial Research. Oral health across the lifespan: children. Available at: https://www.nidcr.nih.gov/research/oralhealthinamerica/section-2-summary. Accessed September 25, 2022.
3. Holve S, Braun P, Irvine JD, et al. Early childhood caries in indigenous communities. *Pediatrics*. 2021;147(6):e2021051481. https://doi.org/10.1542/peds.2021-051481
4. Phipps KR, Ricks TL, Mork NP, Lozon TL. The oral health of American Indian and Alaska Native children aged 1–5 years: results of the 2018–2019 IHS oral health survey. Available at: https://www.ihs.gov/doh/documents/surveillance/2018-19%20Data%20Brief%20of%201-5%20Year-Old%20AI-AN%20Preschool%20Children.pdf. Accessed September 22, 2022.
5. Montana Department of Health and Human Services. The state of the state's oral health. Available at: https://dphhs.mt.gov/assets/ecfsd/OralHealth/OralHealthBurden2020FINAL.pdf. Accessed September 22, 2022.
6. Milgrom P, Weinstein P, Huebner C, Graves J, Tut O. Empowering Head Start to improve access to good oral health for children from low income families. *Matern Child Health J*. 2011;15(7):876–882. https://doi.org/10.1007/s10995-008-0316-6
7. Mathu-Muju KR, Friedman JW, Nash DA. Oral health care for children in countries using dental therapists in public, school-based programs, contrasted with that of the United States, using dentists in a private practice model. *Am J Public Health*. 2013;103(9):e7–e13. https://doi.org/10.2105/AJPH.2013.301251
8. Nash DA, Nagel RJ. Confronting oral health disparities among American Indian/Alaska Native children: the pediatric oral health therapist. *Am J Public Health*. 2005;95(8):1325–1329. https://doi.org/10.2105/AJPH.2005.061796
9. Taylor E, Marino D, Thacker S, DiMarco M, Huff M, Biordi D. Expanding oral health preventative services for young children: a successful interprofessional model. *J Allied Health*. 2014;43(1):e5–e9.
10. Biordi DL, Heitzer M, Mundy E, et al. Improving access and provision of preventive oral health care for very young, poor, and low-income children through a new interdisciplinary partnership. *Am J Public Health*. 2015;105(suppl 2):e23–e29. https://doi.org/10.2105/AJPH.2014.302486
11. Indian Health Service Head Start Program. Classroom circle brushing. Available at: https://www.ihs.gov/HeadStart/documents/ClassroomCircleBrushingPoster.pdf. Accessed September 22, 2022.
12. Northern Cheyenne Tribe. Northern Cheyenne Head Start 2020–2021 annual report. Available at: https://www.cheyennenation.com/index.html. Accessed August 29, 2022.

Statewide Policy to Increase Provision of Take-Home Naloxone at Emergency Department Visits for Opioid Overdose, Rhode Island, 2018–2019

Jennifer Griffith, BA, Rachel R. Yorlets, MPH, Laura C. Chambers, PhD, MPH, Corey S. Davis, JD, MSPH, Anna Wentz, PhD, MPH, Francesca L. Beaudoin, MD, PhD, Janette Baird, PhD, and Elizabeth A. Samuels, MD, MPH, MHS

In 2017, Rhode Island responded to rising overdose deaths by establishing statewide emergency department (ED) treatment standards for opioid overdose and opioid use disorder. One requirement of the policy is that providers prescribe or provide take-home naloxone to anyone presenting to EDs with opioid overdose. Among adults presenting to EDs with opioid overdose from 2018 to 2019, approximately half received take-home naloxone. Receipt of naloxone was associated with administration of naloxone before ED presentation, ED policy certification level, and regional overdose frequency.
(*Am J Public Health*. 2023;113(4):372–377. https://doi.org/10.2105/AJPH.2022.307213)

AJPH April 2023, Vol 113, No. 4

In 2021, more than 107 000 people died of an overdose in the United States, a 15% increase from 2020.[1] With rising overdose deaths, hospitals and emergency departments (EDs) have expanded treatment and harm-reduction services for patients with opioid use disorder (OUD), including distribution of the opioid antagonist naloxone. As a primary treatment site for opioid overdose and OUD, EDs are optimal settings for naloxone distribution and other harm-reduction services.[2]

INTERVENTION AND IMPLEMENTATION

To help standardize and improve ED postoverdose and OUD care, in 2017, the Rhode Island Department of Health (RIDOH) and the Rhode Island Department of Behavioral Healthcare, Developmental Disabilities, and Hospitals established statewide treatment standards for opioid overdose and OUD in EDs and hospitals (known as the "Levels of Care" policy).[3] The policy outlines three levels of certification based on facilities' opioid-related care, with level 1 designating provision of the most comprehensive care and level 3 the minimum treatment standard, and requires all EDs to offer a take-home naloxone kit or naloxone prescription to patients with suspected opioid overdose.[3,4] Previously, ED provision of take-home naloxone was at the discretion of the provider.

RIDOH provided technical assistance to all EDs in Rhode Island to develop and implement protocols in alignment with state policy. This included site visits, review of existing protocols, training of staff, development of patient education materials, and additional implementation support as needed.[5] In the 21 months following policy implementation, 82% of ED patients treated for an opioid overdose were offered take-home naloxone, but less than half received it.[6] While barriers and facilitators to overall policy implementation have been described previously,[5] patient- and facility-level factors influencing provision of take-home naloxone are unknown.

PLACE, TIME, AND PERSONS

Rhode Island has one of the highest rates of overdose death in the United States, ranking 13th in 2020.[7] In 2020, the age-adjusted rate of overdose death was 38.2 deaths per 100 000 residents in Rhode Island (vs 28.3 deaths per 100 000 residents nationally).[7,8]

The ED treatment standards policy was released in March 2017, and ED naloxone distribution protocols were

TABLE 1— Patient Characteristics and Emergency Department Services and Characteristics Among Emergency Department Visits for Opioid Overdose: Rhode Island, 2018–2019

	All Visits (n = 2009), No. (%)	Received Take-Home Naloxone Kit or Naloxone Prescription at Discharge (n = 1170), No. (%)	Did Not Receive Take-Home Naloxone Kit or Naloxone Prescription at Discharge		
			Already Had Naloxone (n = 58), No. (%)	Declined Naloxone (n = 453), No. (%)	Not Offered Naloxone (n = 328), No. (%)
Patient characteristics					
Sex					
Male	1357 (67.5)	805 (68.8)	45 (77.6)	301 (66.4)	206 (62.8)
Female	652 (32.5)	365 (31.2)	13 (22.4)	152 (33.6)	122 (37.2)
Age, y					
18–24	313 (15.6)	180 (15.4)	5 (8.6)	75 (16.6)	53 (16.2)
25–34	811 (40.4)	458 (39.1)	31 (53.4)	193 (42.6)	129 (39.3)
35–44	494 (24.6)	293 (25.0)	15 (25.9)	104 (23.0)	82 (25.0)
45–54	235 (11.7)	145 (12.4)	[a]	45 (9.9)	42 (12.8)
≥ 55	156 (7.8)	94 (8.0)	[a]	36 (7.9)	22 (6.7)
Race					
Black or African American	124 (6.2)	82 (7.0)	[a]	20 (4.4)	21 (6.4)
White	1400 (69.7)	782 (66.8)	51 (87.9)	342 (75.5)	255 (68.6)
Other	69 (3.4)	44 (3.8)	[a]	12 (2.6)	12 (3.7)
Unknown	416 (20.7)	262 (22.4)	5 (8.6)	79 (17.4)	70 (21.3)
Ethnicity					
Hispanic	106 (5.3)	77 (6.6)	[a]	11 (2.4)	15 (4.6)
Non-Hispanic	1122 (55.8)	605 (51.7)	45 (77.6)	285 (62.9)	187 (57.0)
Unknown	781 (38.9)	488 (41.7)	10 (17.2)	157 (34.7)	126 (38.4)
Previous ED visit for opioid overdose in past 12 mo					
Yes	297 (14.8)	167 (14.3)	13 (22.4)	80 (17.7)	37 (11.3)
No	1712 (85.2)	1003 (85.7)	45 (77.6)	373 (82.3)	291 (88.7)
Naloxone administered before ED presentation					
Yes	1671 (83.2)	1005 (85.9)	49 (84.5)	378 (83.4)	239 (72.9)
No	294 (14.6)	141 (12.1)	9 (15.5)	63 (13.9)	81 (24.7)
Unknown	44 (2.2)	24 (2.1)	0 (0.0)	12 (2.6)	8 (2.4)
ED services offered or received					
Offered behavioral counseling					
Yes	1711 (85.2)	1057 (90.3)	52 (89.7)	439 (96.9)	163 (49.7)
No	82 (4.1)	29 (2.5)	[a]	[a]	50 (15.2)
Unknown	216 (10.8)	84 (7.2)	5 (8.6)	12 (2.6)	115 (35.1)
Received behavioral counseling					
Yes	661 (32.9)	542 (46.5)	8 (13.8)	45 (9.9)	66 (20.1)
No	1132 (56.3)	544 (46.5)	45 (77.6)	396 (87.4)	147 (44.8)
Unknown	216 (10.8)	84 (7.2)	5 (8.6)	12 (2.6)	115 (35.1)
Received referral at discharge[b]					
Yes	382 (19.0)	271 (23.2)	9 (15.5)	37 (8.2)	65 (19.8)
No	1627 (81.0)	899 (76.8)	49 (84.5)	416 (91.8)	263 (80.2)

Continued

TABLE 1— Continued

	All Visits (n = 2009), No. (%)	Received Take-Home Naloxone Kit or Naloxone Prescription at Discharge (n = 1170), No. (%)	Did Not Receive Take-Home Naloxone Kit or Naloxone Prescription at Discharge: Already Had Naloxone (n = 58), No. (%)	Declined Naloxone (n = 453), No. (%)	Not Offered Naloxone (n = 328), No. (%)
ED by certification level					
Level 1 (comprehensive care)					
Hospital A	635 (31.6)	428 (36.6)	[a]	111 (24.5)	94 (28.7)
Hospital B	404 (20.1)	143 (12.2)	32 (55.2)	185 (40.8)	44 (13.4)
Hospital C	303 (15.1)	199 (17.0)	5 (8.6)	37 (8.2)	62 (18.9)
Hospital D	176 (8.8)	146 (12.5)	[a]	17 (3.8)	9 (2.7)
Hospital E	55 (2.7)	39 (3.3)	[a]	10 (2.2)	5 (1.5)
Hospital F	39 (1.9)	28 (2.4)	[a]	7 (1.5)	[a]
Level 3 (minimum standard of care)					
Hospital G	266 (13.2)	112 (9.6)	7 (12.1)	64 (14.1)	83 (25.3)
Hospital H	82 (4.1)	46 (3.9)	[a]	8 (1.8)	25 (7.6)
Hospital I	49 (2.4)	29 (2.5)	[a]	14 (3.1)	[a]

Note. ED = emergency department.

[a]Counts of 1–4 are suppressed to prevent potential identification of patients and protect their confidentiality, in accordance with the Rhode Island Department of Health Small Numbers Policy.

[b]Includes referrals to substance use treatment, opioid treatment programs, recovery services, and inpatient detoxification programs.

implemented from March 2017 to June 2018 across all Rhode Island EDs. We evaluated ED distribution of take-home naloxone from nine Rhode Island acute care hospital EDs from January 1, 2018, to December 31, 2019, following policy implementation. Opioid overdose visits to psychiatric and obstetric/gynecologic specialty hospitals were rare and excluded from this analysis.

Our study included all adult patients treated and discharged from a Rhode Island ED after a suspected opioid overdose. Data were obtained from a RIDOH overdose surveillance system to which all Rhode Island EDs are mandated to report suspected opioid overdoses.[9] We excluded patients who were minors, who were incarcerated, who died, who were admitted to the hospital, who left the ED against medical advice, who left without being seen, or who were transferred to another facility.

PURPOSE

The statewide treatment standards aim to improve postoverdose ED care to reduce overdose deaths. Providing take-home naloxone is one component of this strategy. Identifying factors associated with provision of take-home naloxone to ED patients treated for a suspected opioid overdose is essential for improving postoverdose naloxone access.[3]

EVALUATION AND ADVERSE EFFECTS

We aimed to identify patient- and facility-level factors associated with provision of take-home naloxone for ED patients treated after an opioid overdose. From January 1, 2018, to December 31, 2019, 1900 people presented to EDs in Rhode Island for opioid overdose at 2009 unique visits that met inclusion criteria. At more than half of these visits (58.2%; n = 1170) take-home naloxone was provided at discharge, either directly (1110 kits distributed from the ED) or via prescription (60 naloxone prescriptions sent to a pharmacy; Table 1). The primary formulation distributed by hospitals was intranasal.

Among the 1170 visits where naloxone was distributed from the ED, most patients were White (66.8%; n = 782), male (68.8%; n = 805), and aged 25 to 34 years (39.1%; n = 458), as originally recorded in the patient's electronic health record. Among visits where naloxone was not provided (839 visits), more than half declined (54.0%; n = 453), more than a quarter were not offered take-home naloxone (39.1%; n = 328), and a minority reported already having naloxone (6.9%; n = 58).

There were no meaningful differences in patient demographics between different categories of naloxone receipt, and most of our analytic sample was White, male, and young. These demographics reflect the overall composition of people treated in the ED for an opioid overdose.[10] Individuals who died from an opioid overdose had similar race and sex demographic composition but were slightly older compared with the study population (20%–23% of opioid overdose deaths in 2018 and 2019 were among people aged 25 to 34 years).[11,12] Potential explanations for the relatively little diversity found in our analytic sample include limitations of race data recorded in electronic health records, that Rhode Island is a predominantly White state, and potential selection bias in our study because we only included people who were treated in an ED following their opioid overdose.

We fit a multivariable log-binomial regression model specified a priori to estimate the association between patient- and facility-level characteristics and provision of take-home naloxone. Regional frequency of opioid overdose, ED certification level, and administration of naloxone before ED presentation were associated with receipt of take-home naloxone in the ED; these associations were conditional on patient sex, age, race, and whether the patient had a previous ED visit for opioid overdose within the past 12 months (Table 2).

Specifically, patients treated at EDs with a regional frequency of more than 200 emergency medical services (EMS) calls for opioid overdose annually were 1.21 times more likely to receive take-home naloxone in the ED than those treated at EDs with a regional frequency of fewer than 100 opioid overdose EMS calls (95% confidence interval [CI] = 1.10, 1.33). Patients treated at level-1 EDs were 1.18 times more likely to receive take-home naloxone than those at level-3 EDs (95% CI = 1.05, 1.33). Finally, patients who were administered naloxone just before ED arrival were 1.29 times more likely to receive take-home naloxone in the ED than those who were not administered

TABLE 2— Characteristics Associated With Receipt of Take-Home Naloxone at Emergency Department Visits for Opioid Overdose: Rhode Island, 2018–2019

	ED Naloxone Distribution, Adjusted Prevalence Ratio (95% CI)[a]
Sex	
Male	1 (Ref)
Female	0.94 (0.87, 1.02)
Age, y	
18–24	1 (Ref)
25–34	0.93 (0.84, 1.04)
35–44	0.95 (0.85, 1.06)
45–54	1.04 (0.91, 1.19)
≥ 55	0.99 (0.85, 1.15)
Race	
Black or African American	1.04 (0.91, 1.19)
White	1 (Ref)
Other	1.08 (0.91, 1.28)
Unknown	1.00 (0.92, 1.10)
Previous ED visit for opioid overdose in past 12 mo	
Yes	0.94 (0.84, 1.04)
No	1 (Ref)
Naloxone administered before ED presentation	
Yes	1.29 (1.14, 1.46)
No	1 (Ref)
ED certification level	
Level 1 (comprehensive care)	1.18 (1.05, 1.33)
Level 3 (minimum standard of care)	1 (Ref)
Regional frequency of EMS calls for opioid overdose annually	
< 100[b]	1 (Ref)
100–200[c]	0.90 (0.82, 0.99)
> 200[d]	1.21 (1.10, 1.33)

Note. CI = confidence interval; ED = emergency department; EMS = emergency medical services. Multivariable log-binomial regression model fit to n = 1965 ED visits with complete information (97.8% of total study population from Table 1).

[a]Prevalence ratio for ED naloxone distribution. Outcome of ED naloxone distribution collapsed into binary yes/no variable. Model variables included patient characteristics (sex, age, race, ethnicity, ED visit for opioid overdose in past 12 mo, naloxone given before ED arrival), ED certification level (level 1 vs level 3), and annual regional frequency of EMS calls for overdose (< 100, 100–200, > 200).
[b]Barrington, Bristol, Burrillville, Central Falls, Charlestown, Coventry, Cumberland, East Greenwich, East Providence, Exeter, Glocester, Hopkinton, Jamestown, Johnston, Lincoln, Middletown, Narragansett, Newport, North Kingstown, North Providence, North Smithfield, Portsmouth, Richmond, Scituate, Smithfield, South Kingstown, Tiverton, Warren, other, and outside of Rhode Island.
[c]Cranston, Pawtucket, Warwick, Woonsocket, and unknown.
[d]Providence.

naloxone before ED presentation (95% CI = 1.14, 1.46).

There were no known adverse effects or unintended consequences attributable to implementation of the policy or distribution of take-home naloxone in Rhode Island EDs. However, there has not yet been a comprehensive evaluation of ED take-home naloxone receipt to measure its use or other individual outcomes. We identified factors associated with receipt of take-home naloxone at ED visits for opioid overdose in the context of a statewide mandate to offer naloxone to all opioid overdose patients at discharge. This evaluation suggests that additional implementation and training efforts are needed in EDs with a lower certification level (level 3) and in areas that receive fewer than 100 EMS calls for opioid overdose annually. In areas where overdose is treated less frequently, more education and risk awareness are needed among both providers and patients to increase naloxone receipt. Education should also emphasize identifying people at risk for overdose, which includes those who do not receive naloxone before ED arrival.

SUSTAINABILITY

Naloxone for ED distribution is currently purchased by individual hospitals and is not reimbursable, which raises a sustainability concern given rising costs of naloxone[13] and insufficient access to naloxone in the community.[14] Strategies to improve supply, reduce costs of naloxone, and establish insurance reimbursements for naloxone distribution are needed.

PUBLIC HEALTH SIGNIFICANCE

Rhode Island's statewide treatment standards for postoverdose care in EDs aim to improve naloxone access among people at high risk of opioid overdose, with the goal of preventing opioid overdose–related deaths. There are opportunities to improve ED naloxone provision in areas with lower overdose incidence and in EDs with less-comprehensive overdose treatment protocols. Establishing and maintaining a high level of ED naloxone distribution may help to close the naloxone access gaps when community supply is constrained. AJPH

ABOUT THE AUTHORS

Jennifer Griffith is with Brown University, Providence, RI. Rachel R. Yorlets is with the Department of Epidemiology at the Brown University School of Public Health. Laura C. Chambers is with the Substance Use Epidemiology Program at the Rhode Island Department of Health. Corey S. Davis is with the Network for Public Health Law, Edina, MN. Anna Wentz and Francesca L. Beaudoin are with the Department of Epidemiology at the Brown University School of Public Health. Janette Baird and Elizabeth A. Samuels are with the Department of Emergency Medicine at the Warren Alpert Medical School of Brown University.

CORRESPONDENCE

Correspondence should be sent to Elizabeth A. Samuels, MD, MPH, MHS, Associate Professor, Department of Emergency Medicine, University of California, Los Angeles, Los Angeles, CA 90095 (e-mail: lizsamuels@ucla.edu). Reprints can be ordered at https://ajph.org by clicking the "Reprints" link.

PUBLICATION INFORMATION

Full Citation: Griffith J, Yorlets RR, Chambers LC, et al. Statewide policy to increase provision of take-home naloxone at emergency department visits for opioid overdose, Rhode Island, 2018–2019. *Am J Public Health*. 2023;113(4): 372–377.

Acceptance Date: December 15, 2022.

DOI: https://doi.org/10.2105/AJPH.2022.307213

CONTRIBUTORS

L. C. Chambers, C. S. Davis, E. A. Samuels, and R. R. Yorlets contributed to study concept and study design. L. C. Chambers, A. Wentz, and R. R. Yorlets contributed to data extraction. L. C. Chambers and R. R. Yorlets performed data analysis. L. C. Chambers, C. S. Davis, J. Griffith, E. A. Samuels, and R. R. Yorlets interpreted results. J. Griffith, E. A. Samuels, and R. R. Yorlets contributed to initial drafting of the article. All authors contributed to critical revision of the article.

ACKNOWLEDGMENTS

This study was funded by the Centers for Disease Control and Prevention (grants R01CE003149 and NU17CE924967). E. A. Samuels was partially supported by the National Institutes of Health (grants P20GM125507 and U54GM115677) and the Substance Abuse and Mental Health Serrvices Administration (grant UR1TI080209).

The authors would like to acknowledge and thank Jennifier Koziol, MPH, Rachel Scagos, MPH, and the Rhode Island Department of Health Overdose Prevention Program.

Note. The content of this article is solely the responsibility of the authors and does not necessarily represent the official views of the Centers for Disease Control and Prevention, the National Institutes of Health, or the Substance Abuse and Mental Health Services Administration.

CONFLICTS OF INTEREST

The authors have no conflicts of interest to disclose.

HUMAN PARTICIPANT PROTECTION

This study was reviewed and approved by the Lifespan institutional review board.

REFERENCES

1. National Center for Health Statistics. US overdose deaths in 2021 increased half as much as in 2020—but are still up 15%. May 11, 2022. Available at: https://www.cdc.gov/nchs/pressroom/nchs_press_releases/2022/202205.htm. Accessed December 7, 2022.
2. Vivolo-Kantor AM, Seth P, Gladden RM, et al. Vital signs: Trends in emergency department visits for suspected opioid overdoses—United States, July 2016–September 2017. *MMWR Morb Mortal Wkly Rep*. 2018;67(9):279–285. https://doi.org/10.15585/mmwr.mm6709e1
3. Rhode Island Department of Health and Department of Behavioral Healthcare, Developmental Disabilities, and Hospitals. Levels of care for Rhode Island emergency departments and hospitals for treating overdose and opioid use disorder. 2017. Available at: https://health.ri.gov/publications/guides/LevelsOfCareForTreatingOverdoseAndOpioidUseDisorder.pdf. Accessed March 22, 2022.
4. Naloxone effectiveness. A systematic review. *J Addict Nurs*. 2018;29(3):E1–E2. https://doi.org/10.1097/JAN.0000000000000246
5. Samuels EA, McDonald JV, McCormick M, Koziol J, Friedman C, Alexander-Scott N. Emergency department and hospital care for opioid use disorder: implementation of statewide standards in Rhode Island, 2017–2018. *Am J Public Health*. 2019;109(2):263–266. https://doi.org/10.2105/AJPH.2018.304847
6. Samuels EA, Wentz A, McCormick M, et al. Rhode Island's opioid overdose hospital standards and emergency department naloxone distribution, behavioral counseling, and referral to treatment. *Ann Emerg Med*. 2021;78(1):68–79. https://doi.org/10.1016/j.annemergmed.2021.02.004

7. Centers for Disease Control and Prevention. Drug overdose mortality by state. Available at: https://www.cdc.gov/nchs/pressroom/sosmap/drug_poisoning_mortality/drug_poisoning.htm. Accessed December 7, 2022.
8. Hedegaard H, Miniño AM, Spencer MR, Warner M. Drug overdose deaths in the United States, 1999–2020. *NCHS Data Brief.* 2021;(426):1–8.
9. McCormick M, Koziol J, Sanchez K. Development and use of a new opioid overdose surveillance system, 2016. *R I Med J (2013).* 2017;100(4):37–39.
10. Rhode Island Department of Health. Drug Overdose Surveillance Data Hub. Opioid overdose-related emergency department visits. Available at: https://ridoh-drug-overdose-surveillance-eddashboard-rihealth.hub.arcgis.com. Accessed December 7, 2022.
11. PreventOverdoseRI. Overdose death data. Available at: https://preventoverdoseri.org/overdose-deaths. Accessed December 7, 2022.
12. Rhode Island Department of Health. Drug Overdose Surveillance Data Hub. Fatality data: Office of the State Medical Examiners. Available at: https://ridoh-drug-overdose-surveillance-osmedashboard-rihealth.hub.arcgis.com. Accessed December 7, 2022.
13. Gupta R, Shah ND, Ross JS. The rising price of naloxone—risks to efforts to stem overdose deaths. *N Engl J Med.* 2016;375(23):2213–2215. https://doi.org/10.1056/NEJMp1609578
14. Irvine MA, Oller D, Boggis J, et al. Estimating naloxone need in the USA across fentanyl, heroin, and prescription opioid epidemics: a modelling study. *Lancet Public Health.* 2022;7(3):e210–e218. https://doi.org/10.1016/S2468-2667(21)00304-2

Building Broad Public Health Coalitions in the Post-*Roe* World

Alfredo Morabia, MD, PhD

ABOUT THE AUTHOR

Alfredo Morabia is the editor-in-chief of AJPH, *Washington, DC.*

As in every year's April issue of the *Journal*, coinciding with National Public Health Week (#NPHW), we set up a dialogue between people of radically different political views who have in common a dedication to public health and an agreement that policy should be based as much as possible on scientific evidence. The dialogue has covered sensitive issues: racism and structural racism, gun violence prevention, single payer health insurance, public health advocacy, the Environmental Protection Agency, and more (e.g., https://ajph.aphapublications.org/toc/ajph/108/4). This issue is the first to address reproductive rights. It has proven to be the most difficult one to prepare.

The authors of the opinion pieces were invited to comment on the public health consequences of the US Supreme Court's decision to overturn *Roe v Wade* and, in particular, which strategies, at the local and national levels, could best protect pregnant individuals and their children in the new context.

The comments we received, both from progressives and conservatives, stressed the disaster that the decision *Dobbs v Jackson Women's Health Organization* has created for women in this country and beyond.

Frank C. Worrell, PhD, past president of the American Psychological Association, stresses that psychological research shows that the best strategy to prevent mental health issues for women seeking abortions is to make them safe, affordable, and accessible (p. 382).

Kristyn Brandi, MD, MPH, Darney-Landy Fellow at the American College of Obstetricians and Gynecologists, and Puneet Gill, third-year medical student, explain that abortion restrictions will negatively affect the gynecologic profession and the availability of patient care (p. 384).

For Megan Simmons, JD, MPA, policy director of the National Birth Equity Collaborative, and Deneen Robinson, director of religious spiritual policy strategy, National Birth Equity Collaborative, state legislatures codifying abortion rights and access is the best way to ensure bodily autonomy (p. 386).

Herminia Palacio, MD, MPH, president and CEO of the Guttmacher Institute, reminds us that states in which legislators have passed sweeping abortion restrictions concurrently have a terrible track record of promoting health and protecting against preventable maternal, infant, and neonatal deaths (p. 388).

All these comments are consistent with the evidence published in *AJPH* (https://ajph.aphapublications.org/toc/ajph/112/9). However, all of the conservative persons we invited who could be expected to support the Supreme Court decision in one way or another declined to submit or did not even respond.

I therefore asked Sanne Magnan, MD, PhD, senior fellow of the HealthPartners Institute and former Minnesota commissioner of health, to write an opinion editorial. Magnan belongs to a group of the Association of State and Territorial Health Officials alumni, which has been advising for the preparation of the April issues of the *Journal* since 2018. I know she is both dedicated to public health and in favor of alternatives to abortion.

Sanne Magnan is not alone in public health in thinking in these terms, and we need to face this discussion and find, as she insists, "common ground." The cancellation of a federal right to abortion requires broad coalitions to protect reproductive rights in states. Immediate objectives may include preventing unwanted pregnancies using contraception, protecting parents through family and child development policies and Medicaid expansion, and, when possible, avoiding total bans on abortion and the health disasters associated with illegal procedures.

The conclusion of my previous piece titled "Reproductive Rights and Fascist Threat" still reflects my thinking: "Altogether, these [common ground] policies may reduce health inequities and decrease children living in poverty, until the right to abortion and contraception is inserted in the US Constitution."[1(p1229)] AJPH

CORRESPONDENCE

Correspondence should be sent to Alfredo Morabia, MD, PhD, Barry Commoner Center for Health and the Environment, Queens College, CUNY, 65-30 Kissena Blvd, Flushing, NY 11367 (e-mail: amorabia@qc.cuny.edu). Reprints can be ordered at http://www.ajph.org by clicking the "Reprints" link.

PUBLICATION INFORMATION

Full Citation: Morabia A. Building broad public health coalitions in the post-*Roe* world. *Am J Public Health*. 2023;113(4):378–379.

Acceptance Date: February 1, 2023.

DOI: https://doi.org/10.2105/AJPH.2023.307251

CONFLICTS OF INTEREST

The author has no conflicts of interest to declare.

REFERENCE

1. Morabia A. Reproductive rights and fascist threat. *Am J Public Health*. 2022;112(9):1229. https://doi.org/10.2105/AJPH.2022.307001

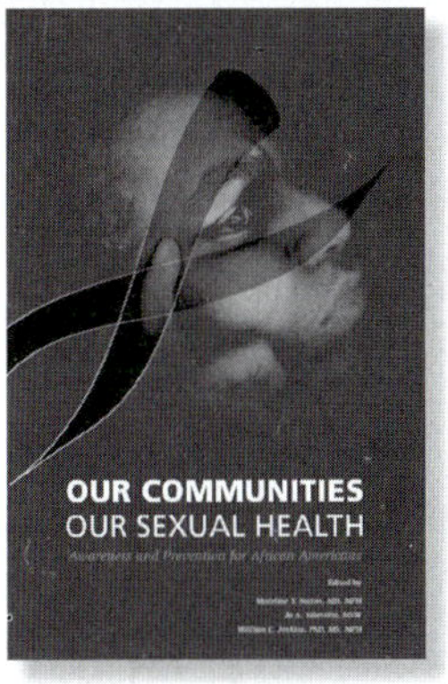

The Potential and Challenges for Common Ground on Abortion

Sanne Magnan, MD, PhD

ABOUT THE AUTHOR

Sanne Magnan is with the HealthPartners Institute, Bloomington, MN.

Note. The opinions expressed in this editorial are solely the author's and do not necessarily reflect the opinions and beliefs of the HealthPartners Institute.

See also Worrell, p. 382, Brandi and Gill, p. 384, Robinson and Simmons, p. 386, and Palacio, p. 388.

Discussing the recent US Supreme Court decision *Dobbs v Jackson Women's Health Organization* (*Dobbs*), a colleague commented, "I am not in favor of abortion, but I don't want to see women in back-street, illegal clinics either." I feel the same way. I understand that women who want abortions advocate reproductive rights; however, who advocates reproductive rights for the unborn? Does it have to be "us" versus "them"? Can we build bridges of empathy for common ground? Can we be a better nation by the process of "listening, asking and understanding"?[1]

To be empathetic[2] is to be curious, get outside our bubbles, and interact with those who do not think as we do. Start with making others feel respected in conversations, even if we do not agree with their positions. Suspend judgments. Acknowledge and explore our privileges and biases. It may lead to shared experiences or understanding differing views on abortion. Is there a shared project, no matter how small, in reproductive rights that could provide a beginning common ground?

Religion is not necessarily a stumbling block for common ground. For example, per the Pew Research Center, the African Methodist Episcopal Church, the Roman Catholic Church, the Southern Baptist Convention, and Hinduism generally oppose abortion rights. The groups on the opposite end of the spectrum (e.g., the Presbyterian Church (USA) and Conservative and Reform Judaism) support abortion rights with few or no limits. There are also religious groups with unclear positions on abortion (e.g., Buddhism, Islam, and Orthodox Judaism).[3] Additionally, individual members may have opinions that do not equate with the official position of their religious group.

An article based on Pew Research Center data has a chart with the heading "85 Percent of American Voters Think Abortion Should Be Legal in Some or All Circumstances."[4] On closer examination, however, this statement is somewhat misleading. The number of people who support legal abortion actually decreases with gestational age. For example, 26% of Americans indicated that abortion should be illegal at the gestational age of six weeks (i.e., illegal with some exceptions, illegal, or illegal in all cases with no exceptions). This number increases to 33% for 14 weeks gestation and 48% for 24 weeks gestation.[4] Therefore, the changing views of Americans on abortion for various stages of gestation may provide fruitful ground for discussion.

But what if seeking common ground on abortion requires uncomfortable listening? On the one hand, there can be the denial of women's bodily autonomy; on the other hand, there can be the denial of the unborn's life—both of which may seem offensive. Finding common ground requires us to listen to each other's rational perspectives, to look for a Venn diagram of next steps. We must start with listening without judgment.

There are two significant challenges for finding common ground: values and views on death and the beginning of life. For example, liberals and conservatives share values such as caring, liberty, and fairness; however, conservatives also tend to embrace others, such as loyalty, authority, and sanctity.[5] Liberty is a key value for advocating women's autonomous decisions about abortion; these reproductive rights are defined from the mother's standpoint: "Who has a right to tell me what to do with my pregnancy and my body?"

Liberty and sanctity are key values for advocating the reproductive rights of the unborn, especially for conservatives, although there is the group Democrats for Life of America (https://www.democratsforlife.org). Underlying sanctity are views on conception and death. Philosopher R. George states, "Each of us who is now an adult is the same human being who was at an earlier time an adolescent, a child, an infant, a fetus, an embryo and a zygote."[6(p191)] Death at any point along this continuum is still death and deprives fetuses of their future life—the good things in life they could have had—if they had lived.[7,8]

Philosopher M. Jali provides another perspective:

AJPH April 2023, Vol 113, No. 4

> It is very difficult to justify any specific time as the point at which a conceptus becomes a person and as such a bearer of moral rights. The pro-life group draws the line as to when the conceptus becomes a person too early. Moderates would find it difficult to accept that a group of cells (regardless of their potentiality) without any form has to be considered as a person. On the other hand, it is also difficult to accept the notion that personhood begins at birth as indicated by the pro-choice group. This view disregard[s] the potentiality towards actual human life that occurs throughout pregnancy.[9(p30)]

Egregious actions after *Dobbs* may spur attention for finding a different way. Criminalizing or creating fear of reprisals in the medical management of spontaneous abortions (i.e., miscarriages), ectopic pregnancies, and noninduced intrauterine fetal death as well as other pregnancy-related issues do not serve either side well and may prompt searches for common ground. On the other hand, introducing legislation with no restrictions on abortion even to the point of birth may be just as egregious.[10,11] However, we could find common ground issues of valuing and investing more in the well-being of our children and families—including in the child tax credit, early childhood education, childcare, and workplace protections for equitable pay, family leave, and suitable medical benefits for pregnant women—ways to support women and families and decrease abortions.[12] Creating the policy environment for such actions will require skillful coalition building, especially in states where such programs have not been supported or funded.

Are these discussions from prolife and prochoice perspectives beneficial for our democracy even if we do not find common ground? Stating and defending beliefs while exploring others' beliefs increase our cognitive capacity. Looking at principles such as justice and equality, we practice our civic duty. Civic care[1] through reasonable disagreements guards against one common perspective becoming entrenched without challenge, decreasing our ability to make good democratic decisions. These disagreements require patience, curiosity, and a willingness to provide a platform for people to be heard. Years from now, will we look back and question whether we created good public policy on abortion?[6] Could slavery in this country have ended earlier if we had done more civic caring?

On November 15, 2022, the *Washington Post's Post Reports* podcast released an episode[13] about the "covert abortion pill pipeline," a pregnant young woman in a loving relationship, her initial ambivalence, and her residence in a state where abortion is illegal. The story is tragic for the impact on her and her pregnancy and best understood by listening to the podcast. In the end, where have we failed this woman and her boyfriend; where have we failed the little one she aborted and they buried? Exploring these questions will not be easy, and building "common ground is not for the faint of heart."[14] AJPH

CORRESPONDENCE

Correspondence should be sent to Sanne Magnan, HealthPartners Institute, Mailstop 21112R, PO Box 1309, Minneapolis, MN 55440-1309 (e-mail: sannemagnan@gmail.com). Reprints can be ordered at http://www.ajph.org by clicking the "Reprints" link.

PUBLICATION INFORMATION

Full Citation: Magnan S. The potential and challenges for common ground on abortion. *Am J Public Health*. 2023;113(4):380–381.

Acceptance Date: February 2, 2023.

DOI: https://doi.org/10.2105/AJPH.2023.307252

CONFLICTS OF INTEREST

The author has no conflicts of interest to disclose.

REFERENCES

1. Miller JP. Caring to disagree: democratic disagreement as civic care. *Polity*. 2012;44(3):400–425. https://doi.org/10.1057/pol.2012.5
2. Miller CC. How to be more empathetic. *New York Times*. January 31, 2019. Available at: https://www.nytimes.com/guides/year-of-living-better/how-to-be-more-empathetic. Accessed January 19, 2023.
3. Masci D. Where major religious groups stand on abortion. June 21, 2016. Available at: https://www.pewresearch.org/fact-tank/2016/06/21/where-major-religious-groups-stand-on-abortion. Accessed January 17, 2023.
4. Molla R. What Americans think about abortions, in 3 charts. June 24, 2022. Available at: https://www.vox.com/policy-and-politics/23167397/abortion-public-opinion-polls-americans. Accessed January 19, 2023.
5. Haidt J. *The Righteous Mind: Why Good People Are Divided by Politics and Religion*. New York, NY: Pantheon Books; 2012.
6. George RP. Democracy and moral disagreement: reciprocity, slavery, and abortion. In: Macedo S, ed. *Deliberative Politics: Essays on Democracy and Disagreement*. New York, NY: Oxford University Press; 1999:184–197.
7. Marquis D. Why abortion is immoral. *J Philos*. 1989;86(4):183–202. https://doi.org/10.2307/2026961
8. Marquis D. Deprivations, futures and the wrongness of killing. *J Med Ethics*. 2001;27(6):363–369. https://doi.org/10.1136/jme.27.6.363
9. Jali MN. Abortion—a philosophical perspective. *Curationis*. 2001;24(4):25–31. https://doi.org/10.4102/curationis.v24i4.878
10. Deng G. Right to abortion bill clears first hurdle in Minnesota House. *Minnesota Reformer*. January 5, 2023. Available at: https://minnesotareformer.com/2023/01/05/right-to-abortion-bill-in-minnesota-clears-first-hurdle. Accessed January 14, 2023.
11. Minnesota Citizens Concerned for Life. Extreme abortion bill passes Minnesota House committee. January 5, 2023. Available at: https://www.mccl.org/post/extreme-abortion-bill-passes-minnesota-house-committee. Accessed January 14, 2023.
12. Koppelman A. The neglected common ground on abortion. *The Hill*. July 17, 2022. Available at: https://thehill.com/opinion/civil-rights/3562469-the-neglected-common-ground-on-abortion. Accessed January 20, 2023.
13. Kitchener C. Inside the covert abortion pill pipeline. *Washington Post*. November 15, 2022. Available at: https://www.washingtonpost.com/podcasts/post-reports/inside-the-covert-abortion-pill-pipeline. Accessed January 18, 2023.
14. Savage S. From frustration to friend: how building common ground made us better. June 15, 2017. Available at: https://www.thindifference.com/2017/06/building-common-ground-made-us-better. Accessed January 10, 2023.

Denying Abortions Endangers Women's Mental and Physical Health

Frank C. Worrell, PhD

ABOUT THE AUTHOR

Frank C. Worrell is the Distinguished Professor in the School of Education at the University of California, Berkeley. He served as the 2022 president of the American Psychological Association.

See also Magnan, p. 380, Brandi and Gill, p. 384, Robinson and Simmons, p. 386, and Palacio, p. 388.

AJPH April 2023, Vol 113, No. 4

State restrictions or outright bans on abortions are putting women's psychological and medical health at risk. Fifty years of psychological research showcase the harmful effects of abortion denial and provide public health leaders with valuable insights on how to promote women's reproductive rights and foster maternal and child health. Key findings from research studies show that, despite claims to the contrary, having an abortion is not linked to mental health problems.

THE LATEST PSYCHOLOGICAL RESEARCH

In a five-year, longitudinal study of more than 1000 women across 21 states, researchers at the University of California, San Francisco, found that those who had abortions were no more likely to report negative emotions, mental health symptoms, or suicidal thoughts than those who were denied an abortion.[1] Five years later, 99% of those who obtained an abortion felt that they had made the right decision, and their most common emotional reaction was relief.

Moreover, women denied abortions have more psychological problems than those who receive them. For example, Biggs et al. found that women who wanted to get an abortion, but were denied one, initially experienced more anxiety symptoms and stress, lower self-esteem, and less life satisfaction than those who received one.[2] Over time, those same women developed more physical health problems than those who received abortions, and two of them later died from complications related to childbirth.[3]

ECONOMIC ISSUES PROMOTING DISTRESS

Women denied abortions also face greater economic hardships. In their summary of research derived from Turnaway Study, the Advancing New Standards in Reproductive Health group at the University of California, San Francisco, noted that women who were denied abortions struggled more financially than those who received an abortion, as evidenced by lower credit scores, more bankruptcies and evictions, and higher poverty rates.[4] These women were also more likely to remain with a violent partner or to raise children alone.

The children of unwanted pregnancies suffer the consequences as well. Because mothers denied abortions are more likely to live in poverty, their children also live in poverty. These children fail to bond well with their mothers, which is connected to poorer outcomes both immediately and later in life.[5] These children also have more social, emotional, and mental health problems over time, and are more likely to be hospitalized for psychiatric problems than their siblings or than children whose pregnancies were planned.[6,7]

Travel for abortion exacts additional psychological and financial tolls. State bans or restrictions on abortion create barriers for those seeking to obtain the procedure. These barriers lead to greater stress, anxiety, and depression, as well as a loss of autonomy—for example, having to tell someone that they were traveling to get the procedure.[8] Indeed, obtaining an abortion is hardest on those with the fewest resources. The new abortion restrictions highlight the harsh reality of health inequities. Women who are least able to access or pay for abortions—those living in poverty, people of color, people in rural areas, sexual and gender minorities, and young people—are most likely to be adversely affected by abortion bans.[9,10]

In sum, psychological research shows the best strategy to prevent mental health issues for women seeking abortions is to make them safe, affordable, and accessible. AJPH

CORRESPONDENCE

Correspondence should be sent to Frank C. Worrell, School Psychology Program, Berkeley School of Education, 2121 Berkeley Way (4th Floor), University of California, Berkeley, CA 94720-1670 (e-mail: frankc@berkeley.edu). Reprints can be ordered at https://ajph.org by clicking the "Reprints" link.

PUBLICATION INFORMATION

Full Citation: Worrell FC. Denying abortions endangers women's mental and physical health. *Am J Public Health.* 2023;113(4):382–383.

Acceptance Date: January 22, 2023.

DOI: https://doi.org/10.2105/AJPH.2023.307241

CONFLICTS OF INTEREST

The author has no conflicts of interest to disclose.

REFERENCES

1. Rocca CH, Samari G, Foster DG, Gould H, Kimport K. Emotions and decision rightness over five years following an abortion: an examination of decision difficulty and abortion stigma. *Soc Sci Med.* 2020;248:112704. https://doi.org/10.1016/j.socscimed.2019.112704
2. Biggs MA, Upadhyay UD, McCulloch CE, Foster DG. Women's mental health and well-being 5 years after receiving or being denied an abortion: a prospective, longitudinal cohort study. *JAMA Psychiatry.* 2017;74(2):169–178. https://doi.org/10.1001/jamapsychiatry.2016.3478
3. Ralph LJ, Schwarz EB, Grossman D, Foster DG. Self-reported physical health of women who did and did not terminate pregnancy after seeking abortion services. *Ann Intern Med.* 2019;171(4):238–247. https://doi.org/10.7326/M18-1666
4. Foster DG, Biggs MA, Ralph L, Gerdts C, Roberts S, Glymour MM. Socioeconomic outcomes of women who receive and women who are denied wanted abortions in the United States. *Am J Public Health.* 2022;112(9):1290–1296. https://doi.org/10.2105/AJPH.2017.304247r
5. Doyle FL, Dickson SJ, Eapen C, et al. Towards preventative psychiatry: concurrent and longitudinal predictors of postnatal maternal–infant bonding. *Child Psychiatry Hum Dev.* 2022; epub ahead of print May 26, 2022. https://doi.org/10.1007/s10578-022-01365-0
6. Dagg PK. The psychological sequalae of therapeutic abortion—denied and completed. *Am J Psychiatry.* 1991;148(5):578–585. https://doi.org/10.1176/ajp.148.5.578
7. David HP. Born unwanted, 35 years later: The Prague Study. *Reprod Health Matters.* 2006;14(27):181–190. https://doi.org/10.1016/S0968-8080(06)27219-7
8. Biggs MA, Kaller S, Ralph L. Barriers accessing abortion care and their association with psychological well-being. *Contraception.* 2020;101(5):355. https://doi.org/10.1016/j.contraception.2020.03.010
9. Kozhimannil KB, Hassan A, Hardeman RR. Abortion access as a racial justice issue. *N Engl J Med.* 2022;387(17):1537–1539. https://doi.org/10.1056/NEJMp2209737
10. Redd SK, Rice WS, Aswani MS, et al. Racial/ethnic and education inequities in restrictive abortion policy variation and adverse birth outcomes in the United States. *BMC Health Serv Res.* 2021;21(1):1139. https://doi.org/10.1186/s12913-021-07165-x

Abortion Restrictions Threaten All Reproductive Health Care Clinicians

Kristyn Brandi, MD, MPH, and Puneet Gill, BA

ABOUT THE AUTHORS

Kristyn Brandi serves as the Darney Landy fellow at the American College of Obstetricians and Gynecologists, Washington, DC. Puneet Gill is a third-year medical student at the College of Osteopathic Medicine, New York Institute of Technology, Old Westbury, NY.

See also Magnan, p. 380, Worrell, p. 382, Robinson and Simmons, p. 386, and Palacio, p. 388.

AJPH April 2023, Vol 113, No. 4

The Supreme Court's decision on *Dobbs v Jackson* will have an impact on reproductive health care provision for years to come, not only where abortion care is now restricted but across the country. As of January 2023, 14 states have outlawed or severely restricted abortion.[1] Morbidity and mortality around the time of labor is already on the rise nationally, from 658 in 2018 to 861 in 2020[2]—particularly in places where abortion is restricted and labor care is increasingly sparse because of loss of the workforce after the COVID-19 pandemic.[3] It is important to understand how the criminalization of abortion providers will affect all other forms of reproductive health care moving forward.

In states where abortion care is currently severely limited, clinicians who provide abortion care face criminalization that can include insurmountable legal fees, loss of their medical license, and even imprisonment. Abortion restrictions create a duality in which providers feel they must serve as agents of the state—reporting any suspicious pregnancy-related issues—or have their license called into question, all while trying to best help their patients. Since these laws took effect, we are already seeing delays in health care services for patients needing early pregnancy care management—for abortion as well as miscarriage management and ectopic pregnancies.[4] Health care providers may be called on to increase surveillance and report signs of abortion that can violate their protection of HIPAA (the Health Insurance Portability and Accountability Act) rights, while also facing malpractice claims if they, by delaying or denying early pregnancy care management, are providing what medical evidence shows to be substandard care.[5]

Beyond losing providers to criminalization, there is the very reasonable reaction that providers may have to these laws, which is to leave their communities and instead provide care in less restrictive states. Many providers are not willing to face the moral injury of restrictive laws preventing them from providing comprehensive, evidence-based care. There are also the potential legal fees providers in states with restrictions will ultimately face, which they may not be able to pay. Thus, some are already leaving their communities to find jobs in states where they can practice without fear or the burden of legal challenges.[6]

It is important to note that providers of abortion care are also providers of other reproductive health care, such as prenatal care, gynecologic services, and gender-affirming care. Communities providers are forced to leave will be left with diminished access to these lifesaving forms of care. This is particularly challenging in rural areas, where there are already scarce prenatal and labor care resources. There is a possibility that providers leaving these communities because of real or perceived risk of criminalization for providing abortion care will result in worse disparities in care for patients overall. This would compound already existing disparities in care in marginalized communities, such as BIPOC (Black, Indigenous, and other people of color), LGBTQI (lesbian, gay, bisexual, transgender/-sexual, queer or questioning, or intersex people), rural areas, those who are incarcerated, those who are undocumented, and those with disabilities.

This is not how health care should work. Health care decisions should be guided by science and evidence, not by politics. Patients will be harmed if providers are forced to choose between their best judgment and their medical license. Communities losing clinicians will lose access to not only abortion care but also other critical reproductive health care. We have an obligation to advocate the reversal of these abortion restrictions and the reestablishment of federal protections so that patients and their doctors can make personal health care decisions that are based in science. AJPH

CORRESPONDENCE

Correspondence should be sent to Kristyn Brandi, MD, MPH, 409 12th St SW, Washington, DC 20024-2188 (e-mail: kbrandi@acog.org). Reprints can be ordered at http://www.ajph.org by clicking the "Reprints" link.

PUBLICATION INFORMATION

Full Citation: Brandi K, Gill P. Abortion restrictions threaten all reproductive health care clinicians. *Am J Public Health*. 2023;113(4):384–385.

Acceptance Date: January 22, 2023.

DOI: https://doi.org/10.2105/AJPH.2023.307239

CONTRIBUTORS

K. Brandi provided the majority of the writing and editing. P. Gill provided background research and editing.

ACKNOWLEDGMENTS

The authors would like to thank the American College of Obstetricians and Gynecologists and Rachel Kingery for their review of this article.

CONFLICTS OF INTEREST

The authors have no conflicts of interest to disclose.

REFERENCES

1. Nash E, Ephross P. State policy trends 2022: in a devastating year, US Supreme Court's decision to overturn Roe leads to bans, confusion and chaos. December 19, 2022. Available at: https://www.guttmacher.org/2022/12/state-policy-trends-2022-devastating-year-us-supreme-courts-decision-overturn-roe-leads. Accessed December 22, 2022.
2. Hoyert DL. Maternal mortality rates in the United States, 2020. *NCHS Health E-Stats*. February 2022. Available at: https://www.cdc.gov/nchs/data/hestat/maternal-mortality/2020/E-stat-Maternal-Mortality-Rates-2022.pdf. Accessed January 28, 2023.
3. Declercq E, Barnard-Mayers R, Zephyrin L, Johnson K. How new state abortion bans and restrictions could worsen access to maternal care and health outcomes. December 2022. Available at: https://www.commonwealthfund.org/publications/issue-briefs/2022/dec/us-maternal-health-divide-limited-services-worse-outcomes. Accessed January 28, 2023. https://doi.org/10.26099/z7dz-8211
4. Arey W, Lerma K, Beasley A, Harper L, Moayedi G, White K. A preview of the dangerous future of abortion bans—Texas Senate Bill 8. *N Engl J Med*. 2022;387(5):388–390. https://doi.org/10.1056/NEJMp2207423
5. Kimport K. Abortion after Dobbs: defendants, denials, and delays. *Sci Adv*. 2022;8(36):eade5327. https://doi.org/10.1126/sciadv.ade5327
6. Noor P. Four months after Roe v Wade was overturned, some providers have left states restricting abortions or changed careers. *The Guardian*. October 26, 2022. Available at: https://www.theguardian.com/world/2022/oct/26/us-abortion-ban-providers-doctors-leaving-states. Accessed December 22, 2022.

Codify Abortion Rights and Access by Way of State Legislatures

Deneen Robinson, BSW, and Megan Simmons, JD, MPA

ABOUT THE AUTHORS

Both authors are with the National Birth Equity Collaborative, Washington, DC.

See also Magnan, p. 380, Worrell, p. 382, Brandi and Gill, p. 384, and Palacio, p. 388.

On June 24, 2022, the US Supreme Court overturned *Roe v Wade*. The ruling in *Dobbs v Jackson Women's Health Organization* (*Dobbs*) essentially left decisions on the legality and accessibility of abortion care in the United States to state legislatures. Furthermore, the holding left to the discretion of states the permissibility of terminating an unintended pregnancy in instances of rape or incest.[1]

Although *Roe v Wade* was often lauded as having legalized abortion, disparities based on race and socioeconomic status have been prevalent since it was passed in 1973. Shortly after the ruling, in 1977, antichoice senator Henry J. Hyde (R, IL) proposed that no federal funds go toward supporting abortion access. The Hyde Amendment barred the use of federal Medicaid funds for abortion except when the life of the person would be endangered by carrying the pregnancy to term. This began the long fight to upend abortion access.

Ironically, states that criminalize and surveil abortion the most stringently, primarily the most religious states, are among the worst states for maternal and infant health outcomes[2]; they often fail to implement adequate and sustainable Medicaid and children's health insurance programs to support the births that have been forced on the pregnant people of these states. People of color, especially Black women, have been disparately affected by this rollback of bodily autonomy couched in the notion of care and concern for the unborn.

CONSEQUENCES

Strains on abortion care facilities were seen almost immediately in states that abut states with some of the most restrictive abortion laws. An influx of women seeking services from neighboring communities increased wait times and put additional pressure on services that were often already sparse. Heartbeat laws, which prohibit an abortion after cardiac activity is detected (which anti-abortion advocates describe as a heartbeat), have complicated medical care, as doctors now hesitate to provide care that was at one time routine and at their medical discretion.

Representative Neal Collins (R, SC), during a public hearing on legislation to ban most abortions, decided not to vote.[3] His concern was prompted by the case of a 19-year-old woman who was 15 weeks pregnant when her water broke. A doctor could not legally extract the fetus because South Carolina had enacted the Fetal Heartbeat Bill (which Representative Collins had voted for). Representative Collins was worried because the doctor told him the young woman had a "50 percent chance of losing her uterus, and there was a 10 percent chance she would develop sepsis and die."[3]

The ramifications of abortion restrictions are particularly problematic in the South, where many states with the most restrictive laws are located and border each other. These facts make it difficult to obtain abortion care because an individual has to travel through more than one state to reach a medical facility. This is particularly a hardship for Black women, as 56% of Black people live in the South.[4] Furthermore, Black women are disparately affected by wage and economic inequality, which impedes access to child care, transportation, leave from work, and out-of-town accommodations. Discussions about self-managed abortions have become more prevalent and are a realistic option when reproductive rights have been inhibited.

Financial constraints account for most decisions to terminate a pregnancy.[5] In an amicus brief filed on behalf of the respondents in *Dobbs*, 154 economists said, "A substantial body of well-developed and credible research" shows that abortion legalization and access has had a significant impact on women's educational attainment and wages, "with impacts most strongly felt by Black women."[6] Restrictions on bodily autonomy subjugate women and solidify them as a permanent economic underclass. Although this may align with the religious sensibilities of those in power in our country, it does not support the desires of women to be full citizens experiencing full bodily autonomy.

AJPH April 2023, Vol 113, No. 4

The legal inconsistencies from making abortion a state issue have made it more cumbersome to educate constituents on accessibility options. Navigating this rollback of individual rights requires advocates to simultaneously know about developing solutions that are actionable, such as the creation of mobile abortion clinics on state borders and fundraising for abortions services; facilitate outreach; and demand statutes that are auxiliaries to abortion, such as telemedicine options (which are particularly beneficial in rural communities), and the revocation of laws that encourage medical surveillance and mandates for physicians to report legally obtained abortions.

STRATEGIES TO PROTECT WOMEN AND CHILDREN

On January 5, 2023, the South Carolina Supreme Court held that the state constitution provides the right to privacy, which includes the right to obtain an abortion.[4] There have been approximately 19 lawsuits that have been filed in other states to codify the right to abortion care. Given this intrusion and revocation of rights, the most optimal strategic plan is for state legislatures to codify abortion rights and access. The laws' language should be clear and concise to ensure that it is interpreted to protect bodily autonomy without overreach and interruption from the government. Concurrently, stakeholders should continue to work toward policies that support access to the full range of reproductive care for all people with the capacity to become pregnant, including broadband accessibility; workplace protections for leave, pay equity, and suitable medical benefits; and regulations that support equitable maternal health and education. AJPH

CORRESPONDENCE

Correspondence should be sent to Megan Simmons, Policy Director, National Birth Equity Collaborative, 1301 Connecticut Ave NW, Suite 200, Washington, DC 20026 (e-mail: mrsimmonsjd@gmail.com). Reprints can be ordered at http://www.ajph.org by clicking the "Reprints" link.

PUBLICATION INFORMATION

Full Citation: Robinson D, Simmons M. Codify abortion rights and access by way of state legislatures. *Am J Public Health*. 2023;113(4):386–387.

Acceptance Date: January 23, 2023.

DOI: https://doi.org/10.2105/AJPH.2023.307238

CONTRIBUTORS

Both authors drafted and revised the article.

CONFLICTS OF INTEREST

The authors have no known conflicts of interest.

REFERENCES

1. *Dobbs v. Jackson Women's Health Organization*, docket no. 19-1392 (June 24, 2022). Available at: https://www.supremecourt.gov/opinions/21pdf/19-1392_6j37.pdf. Accessed February 1, 2023.
2. Landi H. In states with abortion bans, maternal and infant death rates are significantly higher, study finds. December 14, 2022. Available at: https://www.fiercehealthcare.com/providers/states-abortion-bans-maternal-and-infant-death-rates-are-dramatically-higher-study-finds. Accessed February 1, 2023.
3. Patterson C. S.C. rep. who voted for abortion restriction shares emotional account of teen affected: "that weighs on me." August 23, 2022. Available at: https://people.com/health/south-carolina-rep-who-voted-for-abortion-restriction-shares-emotional-account-of-teen-affected. Accessed February 1, 2023.
4. Zernike K. South Carolina constitution includes abortion right, state supreme court rules. *New York Times*. January 5, 2023. Available at: https://www.nytimes.com/2023/01/05/us/south-carolina-abortion-supreme-court.html. Accessed February 1, 2023.
5. Foster DG, Biggs MA, Ralph L, Gerdts C, Roberts S, Glymour MM. Socioeconomic outcomes of women who receive and women who are denied wanted abortions in the United States. *Am J Public Health*. 2018;108(3):407–413. https://doi.org/10.2105/AJPH.2017.304247
6. Brief of Amici Curiae Economists in Support of Respondents. *Dobbs v. Jackson Women's Health Organization*, docket no. 19-1392 (September 20, 2021). Available at: https://www.supremecourt.gov/DocketPDF/19/19-1392/193084/20210920175559884_19-1392bsacEconomists.pdf. Accessed February 1, 2023.

Implications of *Dobbs v Jackson Women's Health Organization*

Herminia Palacio, MD, MPH

ABOUT THE AUTHOR

Herminia Palacio is with the Guttmacher Institute, New York, NY.

See also Magnan, p. 380, Worrell, p. 382, Brandi and Gill, p. 384, and Robinson and Simmons, p. 386.

During its consideration of *Dobbs v Jackson Women's Health Organization*, the US Supreme Court received several scientifically, medically, and ethically sound amicus briefs in strong opposition to Mississippi's abortion ban. Among those briefs was one that stated clearly and succinctly that "abortion is a safe, common, and essential component of healthcare." This amicus brief was submitted jointly by the nation's leading medical professional membership organizations: the American College of Obstetricians and Gynecologists, the American Medical Association, the American Association of Public Health Physicians, the American Academy of Family Physicians, the American Academy of Nursing, and the American Academy of Pediatrics.[1] The abundance of compelling evidence notwithstanding, on June 24, 2022, the Supreme Court issued its ruling in *Dobbs*, overturning 50 years of a federally protected right to abortion services while simultaneously telegraphing, through a concurring opinion written by Justice Clarence Thomas, that "all of this Court's substantive due process precedents" should be up for reconsideration.

Six months later, what are the realized and potential consequences, especially as they relate to maternal health outcomes? As of January 1, 2023, the Guttmacher Institute has categorized 26 states as having restrictive abortion policies.[2] Many of the abortion-restrictive states are geographically contiguous, further extending the travel distance required for residents of some states to obtain a legal abortion in another state.[2] This also has the potential to create regions in the country where health care providers are unable to learn basic skills in providing abortion care, which can have ripple effects on the workforce and quality of abortion care nationally.

A recent analysis identified differences in maternal and neonatal outcomes by state abortion policy category.[3] Compared with the District of Columbia and the 24 states where abortion is more accessible,[2,3] states with restrictive policies had fewer maternity health care resources, higher maternal mortality rates, and higher infant and perinatal mortality rates.[3] Taken together, these results highlight a troubling reality: the very same states in which legislators have passed sweeping abortion restrictions concurrently have a terrible track record of promoting health and protecting against preventable maternal, neonate, and older infant deaths. And although such adverse consequences continue to be disproportionately experienced by people of color in both abortion-restricted and abortion-accessible states, when the authors applied the Commonwealth Fund health equity health system performance scorecard, they found more equitable outcomes in abortion-accessible states.[3]

Evidence continues to demonstrate that access to abortion services is an important tool for promoting maternal health. A recent study of women with pregnancy complications before 22 weeks' gestation found that 57% who underwent state-mandated expectant management experienced a serious maternal morbidity, compared with 33% who chose an abortion under similar clinical circumstances in states without such a mandate.[4] As this study shows, such policy approaches do not improve maternal health but may actually worsen it. To better protect pregnant individuals and children, states have an urgent need to repeal abortion restrictions. But that is not enough. They must also direct increased resources to improving maternal and child care and to eliminating inequities in access and outcomes.

Although these policies play out on a state-by-state basis, at the federal level, even after the *Dobbs* decision, Congress has not yet managed to pass either the Women's Health Protection Act[5] or the Equal Access to Abortion Coverage in Health Insurance Act.[6]

I have focused on the potential impact of the *Dobbs* decision on maternal and neonatal outcomes; however, I must circle back to the ominous concurring opinion of Justice Thomas. The 117th Congress partially took him at his word—and it passed, and President Biden signed, the Respect for Marriage Act, which protects same-sex marriage and interracial marriage.[7,8] Nevertheless, the assaults on abortion care via state

AJPH April 2023, Vol 113, No. 4

legislation and regulation continue,[9] as do the assaults on gender-affirming care.[10]

"Public health is what we, as a society, do collectively to assure the conditions in which people can be healthy."[11(p1)] Protecting the full scope of sexual and reproductive health and rights, and doing so in a manner that accelerates and ensures equity and justice, are imperative components of what we, as a society, must do collectively. AJPH

CORRESPONDENCE

Correspondence should be sent to Herminia Palacio, MD, MPH, President, CEO, Guttmacher Institute, 125 Maiden Ln, 7th Floor, New York, NY 10038 (e-mail: hpalacio@guttmacher.org). Reprints can be ordered at http://www.ajph.org by clicking the "Reprints" link.

PUBLICATION INFORMATION

Full Citation: Palacio H. Implications of *Dobbs v Jackson Women's Health Organization*. *Am J Public Health*. 2023;113(4):388–389.

Acceptance Date: January 22, 2023.

DOI: https://doi.org/10.2105/AJPH.2023.307244

CONFLICTS OF INTEREST

The author has no conflicts of interest to declare.

REFERENCES

1. Brief of American College of Obstetricians and Gynecologists, et al. *Dobbs v. Jackson Women's Health Organization* (2021). Available at: https://www.supremecourt.gov/DocketPDF/19/19-1392/193074/20210920174518042_19-1392%20bsacACOGetal.pdf. Accessed January 5, 2023.
2. Guttmacher Institute. Interactive map: US abortion policies and access after Roe. January 2023. Available at: https://states.guttmacher.org/policies. Accessed January 7, 2023.
3. Declercq E, Barnard-Mayers R, Zephyrin L, Johnson K. The US maternal health divide: the limited maternal health services and worse outcomes of states proposing new abortion restrictions. December 14, 2022. Available at: https://www.commonwealthfund.org/publications/issue-briefs/2022/dec/us-maternal-health-divide-limited-services-worse-outcomes. Accessed January 7, 2023.
4. Nambiar A, Patel S, Santiago-Munoz P, Spong CY, Nelson DB. Maternal morbidity and fetal outcomes among pregnant women at 22 weeks' gestation or less with complications in 2 Texas hospitals after legislation on abortion. *Am J Obstet Gynecol*. 2022;227(4):648–650.e1. https://doi.org/10.1016/j.ajog.2022.06.060
5. Congress.gov. HR 3755—Women's Health Protection Act of 2021. 117th Congress (2021–2022). Available at: https://www.congress.gov/bill/117th-congress/house-bill/3755/text. Accessed January 7, 2023.
6. Congress.gov. HR 1692—Equal Access to Abortion Coverage in Health Insurance (EACH Woman) Act of 2019. 116th Congress (2019–2020). Available at: https://www.congress.gov/bill/116th-congress/house-bill/1692. Accessed January 7, 2023.
7. American Presidency Project. President Biden signs the Respect for Marriage Act. December 14, 2022. Available at: https://www.presidency.ucsb.edu/documents/what-they-are-saying-president-biden-signs-the-respect-for-marriage-act. Accessed January 7, 2023.
8. Congress.gov. HR 8404—Respect for Marriage Act. 117th Congress (2021–2022). Available at: https://www.congress.gov/bill/117th-congress/house-bill/8404/text. Accessed January 7, 2023.
9. Nash E, Ephross P. In a devastating year, US Supreme Court's decision to overturn Roe leads to bans, confusion and chaos. December 19, 2022. Available at: https://www.guttmacher.org/2022/12/state-policy-trends-2022-devastating-year-us-supreme-courts-decision-overturn-roe-leads. Accessed January 7, 2023.
10. Migdon B. Here are the states planning to restrict gender-affirming care next year. December 29, 2022. Available at: https://thehill.com/changing-america/respect/diversity-inclusion/3789757-here-are-the-states-planning-to-restrict-gender-affirming-care-next-year. Accessed January 7, 2023.
11. Institute of Medicine. *The Future of Public Health*. Washington, DC: National Academies Press; 1988.

The First Publication on Contraception in a US Medical Journal, 1928: Hannah Mayer Stone's Case for Contraceptive Care Before the Pill

Robin E. Jensen, PhD

Today, as access to women's reproductive health care in the United States has proven less than ensured, it behooves scholars of public health to explore how US medical contraceptive care was successfully established and perpetuated initially in the early to mid-twentieth century. This article highlights the work of Hannah Mayer Stone, MD, in building and advocating such care. From the moment she accepted the position of medical director for the first contraceptive clinic in the country in 1925 until her untimely death in 1941, Stone campaigned relentlessly for women's access to the best contraceptive regimes available, all the while navigating extensive legal, social, and scientific challenges. In 1928, she published the first scientific report on contraception in a US medical journal, thereby legitimating the provision of contraception as a medical endeavor and providing empirical grounds for clinical contraceptive work in the years that followed. Her scientific publications and professional correspondence provide insight into the processes through which medical contraceptive care became increasingly available in US history and offer guidance for a contemporary era when reproductive health care hangs in the balance. (*Am J Public Health*. 2023;113(4):390–396. https://doi.org/10.2105/AJPH.2022.307215)

AJPH April 2023, Vol 113, No. 4

The story of US women gaining access to safe and effective contraception is one that often focuses on major technological advancements, such as the development of the birth control pill.[1] Yet, long before the pill went on the market in the 1960s, a network of medical contraceptive care prescribing largely female-controlled contraceptive devices and products had already been established.[2] Hannah Mayer Stone, MD, (Figure 1) played a central role in building the empirical foundation for that care in the 1920s and '30s. Today, in an era when access to effective contraception is more imperative than it has been in the last 50 years, it behooves scholars of public health to identify the processes through which contraceptive care was made increasingly available in US history, particularly as those processes unfolded alongside the accumulation of medical knowledge about developing birth control technologies.

In 1928, Stone authored the first report on contraception ever published in a US medical journal, in the *Medical Journal and Record*.[3] Just three years before, she had agreed to become medical director of the country's first legal contraceptive clinic, the Clinical Research Bureau of the American Birth Control League (later renamed the Birth Control Clinical Research Bureau), directed by Margaret Sanger and located in downtown New York City. At that point, there were scarce scientific data concerning the safety or efficacy of available contraceptives.

It was only in 1918 that—in the state of New York—physicians alone were granted the right to discuss or prescribe contraceptives at all,[4] but this right was of limited value without associated medical information concerning which methods worked and under what circumstances. To address this problem, Stone coupled her in-depth consultations at the clinic with meticulous record-keeping about patients' experiences with specific contraceptive regimes. Overall, she collaborated with patients to collect almost 100 000

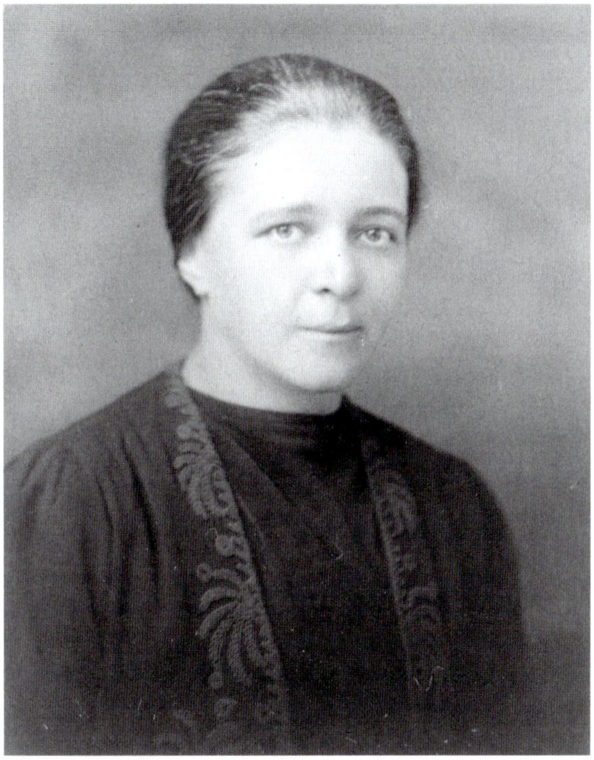

FIGURE 1— Hannah Mayer Stone, MD

Note. This photo was taken between 1930 and 1940.
Source. Property of the Harvard Medical Library collection, Center for the History of Medicine in the Francis A. Countway Library of Medicine. Printed with permission.

contraceptive case histories before her untimely death in 1941.[5] Her 1928 publication was based on the earliest of these histories and reveals that Stone's patients themselves—in undergoing examination and study enrollment—played a vital role in shaping subsequent medical practice.

Drawing from a selection of Stone's scientific publications and archived professional correspondence, this article explores how Stone managed to practice medicine and perform foundational research despite a hostile legal and social climate. By translating her patients' individualized case histories into published medical data and fostering a professional network of data sharing and collaboration, Stone made it increasingly possible for health care providers, herself included, to offer the kind of empirically based care that best fit individuals' specific circumstances and facilitated desired outcomes. Given the parallels between Stone's provision of individualized birth control in the 1920s and recent calls concerning the need for such care among underserved and marginalized patients in particular in 2022,[6] I argue that Stone's research and interprofessional advocacy offer contemporary providers guidance for navigating the contested landscape of current US reproductive health care and social justice.

CHALLENGES TO EARLY CONTRACEPTIVE CARE

Extensive challenges stood in the way of efforts to establish safe and effective contraceptive care in the early twentieth century. Beginning in 1873, Comstock laws went into effect that categorized all contraceptive information and products as obscene and therefore as illegal to possess or send through the US mail.[7] When birth control advocate Margaret Sanger first tried to establish a contraceptive clinic in 1916 that was modeled on clinics in the Netherlands, her clinic was raided by police and shut down under the Comstock laws.

In 1918, the New York State Court of Appeals made a provision for licensed physicians specifically to prescribe contraception to married couples for the prevention or cure of disease, which the judge interpreted broadly to include any change in the body that could disturb health.[8] In accordance with this ruling, Sanger re-established her contraceptive clinic in 1923 with a licensed physician at the helm. Sanger first hired Dorothy Bocker, MD, to serve as medical director, but she dismissed Bocker two years later for failure to keep adequate records and hired Stone as her replacement. At the time, Stone was a practicing physician at New York City's Lying-In Hospital who was trained in pharmacology and shared a joint practice with her husband, the urologist Abraham Stone, MD.

Stone originally met Sanger when she attended the first national birth control conference in 1921 and expressed interest in the emergent birth control movement. In her role as medical director, Stone turned the clinic into something of an "über-clinic" that offered clinical care and generated empirical data about contraceptives.[9] Her research provided other clinics being established across the country and internationally with the statistical and qualitative data needed to prescribe the most effective medical contraceptive care available.

This was the case even as contraceptive care providers continued to struggle for years to offer services within the bounds of an unfavorable legal backdrop. Although Sanger and Stone would win the right for physicians to send and receive contraceptives through the US mail in 1936 in *US v. One Package*,[10] it was not until 1965 that the Supreme Court established the federal right to contraception for married couples, 1972 that it granted the right to contraception for unmarried individuals, and 1977 that it found unconstitutional all restrictions on the advertising, selling, or distributing of contraception.[11]

Throughout the twentieth century, legal barriers to establishing contraceptive care were compounded by associated social and professional challenges. As Sanger recalled of the 1920s, "few doctors wanted to take the risk of identifying themselves with the birth control cause, the risk of becoming a martyr, of losing professional license or standing, of being expelled from their medical societies."[12] As it happened, all of these fates befell Stone, who—as one of very few female practicing physicians at the time—had already experienced significant marginalization and discrimination throughout her early career. Upon signing on as medical director, a position for which she never accepted remuneration,[13] Stone was dismissed from her position at the Lying-In Hospital, blocked from professional societies, and shunned by former colleagues.[14]

When she was attempting to publish her scientific findings on contraception, her professional correspondence provides evidence of the rejection she faced. In a letter from 1925, the editor of the *Medical Journal and Record* (the same outlet that eventually published her work three years later under a different editor) reported, "I have made inquiries regarding the publication of articles on birth control, and I regret to be obliged to return your manuscript on 'Contraceptive Methods of Choice,' as our Journal would be unmailable with this article included."[15] Other letters illustrate that this type of professional rebuff reverberated into the public sphere as well. In 1937, a radio station's legal counselor informed Stone that the station did "not wish to jeopardize its license from the Federal Communications Commission" to broadcast an address she was to give on contraception.[16] At every turn, Stone's ability to circulate her findings and facilitate care was hampered, sometimes publicly, but more often via interactions outside public view.

The legal and professional hardships that Stone encountered also overlapped with challenges posed at the levels of science and medical inquiry. When Stone began her directorship, there was inadequate scientific data to guide clinical contraceptive care. Several physicians from this time spoke to this effect, including practitioners such as Robert L. Dickinson, MD. As a renowned gynecologist in his own right and director of the at-times-competing Committee on Maternal Health,[17] Dickinson's assessment held weight. In his introduction to Stone's 1928 medical publication, he explained:

> the library of argument and invective on the subject of birth control was built on an absurdly small amount of medical information. At that time the Committee on Maternal Health did not find over thirty cases, properly accredited and followed up, on which to start clinical studies. The gynecological and obstetrical departments of medical colleges have been reluctant to bestir themselves in accumulating records of cases requiring contraceptive advice for the safeguarding of life and health.[18]

Without existing data to consult, Stone gathered, analyzed, and presented her own data from the clinic's patients to begin establishing contraceptive care as an empirically based pursuit.[19]

TRANSLATING WOMEN'S EMBODIED EXPERIENCES INTO EMPIRICAL DATA

In a remembrance of Stone delivered in 1941, Sanger said of her that "no one, certainly, has more thoroughly explored the clinical aspects of contraception."[20] Long before the first randomized controlled trials, Stone oversaw and administered the country's first large-scale clinical study of contraception by documenting her patients' experiences with specific contraceptive regimes and compiling these considerable data into scientific reports. When she published one report in a US medical journal in 1928, she initiated the broader process of validating contraceptive care among US physicians by providing them with the empirical evidence needed to offer such care and delivering it in a professionally recognized outlet.

At that point, contraception had been rejected by polite society and physicians alike as the stuff of immorality and vice,[21] and the task of legitimizing contraception as part of standard US medical practice remained far from complete until well into the 1970s.[22] Stone's 1928 publication helped to begin the long process of situating birth control culturally as aboveboard and within the expertise of authorized medical practitioners. Given it was only physicians who had the legal ability to council on and prescribe contraception, their eventual willingness to perceive birth control care as a legitimate part of their work was the pivot upon which the US birth control movement rested for much of the twentieth century.

Stone's 1928 article performed its legitimacy by detailing how she designed her patient consultations to support a rigorous statistical study of available contraceptive regimes (Figure A, available as a supplement to the online version of this article at https://ajph.org). Stone explained that she reduced potential biases in design through extraordinary efforts that included overseeing every one of the 1655 patient consultations herself (with multiple consultations across patients) and performing the consultations over the same period (1925–1927). She described instituting a system of record keeping that allowed her to detail each aspect of her study design including the specific type of contraceptive regimen each participant was prescribed (primarily different formulas of spermicidal jellies combined with occlusive pessaries), exact chemical content of jellies employed, processes involved in measuring and fitting pessaries and diaphragms, precise instructions participants received during initial and follow-up consultations, period of adherence, qualitative feedback, and regime outcome. She noted, "each patient was asked to return at certain intervals, or else to report by mail the results with the method prescribed."[23] Stone's report highlighted her efforts to obtain comprehensive information about the contraceptive experiences of as many women as possible.

Above all else, Stone's article contended that effective contraceptive care must be personalized and attendant to every patient's unique body, circumstances, and experiences, and not just because pessaries and diaphragms required medical fittings. Scattered throughout Stone's numeric findings are notations about how "each patient was examined individually, and a contraceptive chosen according to the needs and indications of the particular case,"[24] and reminders that "much tact and care must be employed in obtaining reports from patients. The use of contraceptives is a very intimate problem with the woman."[25] She reported that some patients found specific regimens uncomfortable, physically irritating, or requiring of more privacy than they had available. Stone upheld these responses as valid reasons for regime noncompliance and therefore as issues for other physicians to anticipate in their own consultations.

In her conclusion, Stone made recommendations about which contraceptive regimes were most effective. But rather than recommending the most statistically effective regimen across the board (a Ramses-type pessary with "Formula I" jelly), she endorsed a different regime (a Ramses-type pessary with "Formula V" jelly) for many cases because some patients reported "trouble" with the former.[26] In this way, Stone modeled how to balance statistical findings with qualitative patient feedback.

ESTABLISHING A SYSTEM OF COLLECTIVE PRACTICES

Although Stone composed the earliest of her reports from her own patient consultations alone, she knew the long-term establishment of robust contraceptive care would require incorporation of more diverse data and the explicit sharing of clinical information and experiences across contexts and demographics. Stone's work to foster a network of contraceptive care knowledge was less visible than her clinical research because it was initiated largely behind the scenes. Beginning as early as 1927, Stone contacted physicians who were "actively engaged in contraceptive work" across the country and internationally to provide overviews of her data and the clinic's contraceptive resources. She distributed surveys asking them to share their emergent contraceptive insights, promising "due credit" for those "willing to contribute" to future reports.[27] In a letter from 1933, she explained:

> We hope that this questionnaire may serve to develop a more regular exchange of information and data among the various clinics in this country. . . . We shall be glad to supply information on any of the methods which we have already tested, and to investigate in the laboratory any newer methods that other clinics might be interested in.[28]

Additional correspondence, along with the more comprehensive evidence included in her subsequent medical reports, revealed that Stone's efforts to foster cooperative values were fruitful. In a 1935 letter addressed to a physician in Florida, for instance, Stone wrote, "I was very much pleased to receive your application blanks and to know that you are willing to cooperate with us in our new project," before noting, "Our aim is to be mutually helpful in developing the practice of contraception and we shall, no doubt, find many occasions in the future to exchange data, findings and information."[29] Stone's correspondence also revealed that she started a "Printed Matter Exchange" so that providers would not have to create materials from scratch

AJPH April 2023, Vol 113, No. 4

and could compare their processes and procedures with other clinics.[30]

In addition, Stone's correspondence demonstrated that she fostered collaboration by interacting one on one with other physicians concerning the ins and outs of contraceptive care. In some instances, Stone had to forgo niceties to critique others' regimes or products. In 1935, she wrote to a collaborating physician, "The jelly which you sent us, which is made up from the Dupont product, I found to be too irritating. Women complained of burning and irritation very soon after the insertion of the jelly. It is likely that the percentage is too strong, or that irritation could be obviated by changes in the form of manufacture."[31] In a 1938 correspondence with Dickinson, she explained that a series of trials she conducted revealed that a particular pessary's "construction of its rim makes it too stiff and apt to cause too much pressure," concluding that "it still requires a certain amount of technical improvement."[32] Stone coupled calls for cooperation with a willingness to engage honestly about what would serve individuals' needs best, drawing from patient feedback as evidence for objections. If she found existing products and regimes unsatisfactory, she called for collaborative efforts to make improvements.

Moreover, for Stone, persuading others to collaborate involved demonstrating that she, too, would meet individual patients where they were and provide them with what they needed. She regularly responded—via letter and often with requested materials such as medical directories—to women who were desperate for contraceptive information.[33] She gave them sometimes lengthy, always personalized advice and encouraged them not to "hesitate to write again at any time we can be of any help."[34] Stone's care for individuals led her to send contraceptive supplies to, in one case, a woman in Barranquilla, Colombia, who wrote her and was without access.[35] In this way, she modeled her belief that personalized, direct engagement was imperative for providing contraceptive care that would work in any given case.

CONTRACEPTIVE CARE TODAY

Today, much can be garnered from Stone's record of contraceptive care advocacy. Comparatively, the good news is that contemporary providers and public health advocates are facing different, and arguably fewer, headwinds than did Stone in their fight to create and sustain safe and effective contraceptive care. Unlike in Stone's time, there exists vast scientific, empirical evidence about contraceptive uses, outcomes, and risks across a variety of circumstances and demographics, evidence that is generated by pharmaceutical companies rather than already overtaxed practicing physicians. Moreover, contraceptive methods today are more varied, available, and effective. Yet, there are still significant obstacles to providing reproductive health care in the twenty-first century. These involve factors such as evolving federal and state legislative restrictions, inadequate clinical guidelines and training, vast health care–access inequities and biases, and a lack of "person-centered approaches" to contraceptive care.[36]

Given that contraceptive care remains precarious, Stone's approach to providing and advocating care in a fraught reproductive health climate offers guidance for today. First, even in contexts in which generating statistical results was necessary, Stone saw that her patients' embodied experiences with contraceptive regimes were accounted for. She argued that effective care depends on personalized engagement with patients as much as on prescribing methods grounded in statistical outcomes. To highlight the importance of finding this balance, she included in her 1928 statistical report references to the embodied experiences of individuals in her care, and she incorporated specific ideas generated from those references in making recommendations about prescribed contraceptive regimes. Stone did so to such an extent that the integral role clinic patients themselves played in shaping subsequent medical practice becomes clear.

Today's physicians do not need to prove contraceptive regime effectiveness as Stone did, but the success of their work depends no less on individualized, patient-centered clinical care and contraceptive counseling. Such an approach, grounded in listening and dedicated attention to patients' unique situations and positionalities, aligns with efforts to foster reproductive justice. A reproductive justice framework centers individuals' intersectional identities considering systemic inequalities to provide increasingly safe, effective, and equitable care.[37] It involves upholding patient experiences and histories as agentic, as did Stone, and illuminating hard truths related to, for instance, the history of coercion and deception employed against Black, Latinx, and Indigenous individuals by medical authorities in the context of US contraceptive care.[38]

Second, Stone's work involved advocating a system of sharing and collaboration among fellow physicians. She built bridges, speaking and acting in ways that emphasized cooperation and a mutual vision. Her surviving professional correspondence reveals how she initiated large-scale campaigns that involved sharing information among contraceptive care providers. It also reveals her efforts to engage openly with other providers about patient experiences. Throughout her career, Stone made it clear that the effective provision of contraceptive care always starts and stops with attention to the experiences and needs of individual patients. In the twenty-first century, as in the early twentieth, there can be no more important lesson to be taken from her body of work. AJPH

ABOUT THE AUTHOR

Robin E. Jensen is a professor in the Department of Communication, University of Utah, Salt Lake City.

CORRESPONDENCE

Correspondence should be sent to Robin E. Jensen, PhD, Department of Communication, University of Utah, 255 S Central Campus Drive, Salt Lake City, UT 84112 (e-mail: r.e.jensen@utah.edu). Reprints can be ordered at https://ajph.org by clicking the "Reprints" link.

PUBLICATION INFORMATION

Full Citation: Jensen RE. The first publication on contraception in a US medical journal, 1928: Hannah Mayer Stone's case for contraceptive care before the pill. *Am J Public Health*. 2023; 113(4):390–396.

Acceptance Date: December 15, 2022.

DOI: https://doi.org/10.2105/AJPH.2022.307215

ACKNOWLEDGMENTS

Funding for this study was provided by a National Endowment for the Humanities Faculty Fellowship (FEL-267498-20).

I am grateful to archivists Kate Long and Maureen Callahan at Smith College's Special Collections, as well as archivist Stephanie Krauss at the Center for the History of Medicine in the Francis A. Countway Library of Medicine at Harvard University, for helping me to obtain access to the materials cited in this essay. Many thanks, also, are extended to the editor and four anonymous reviewers for their engagement and dedication to this research.

Note. Any views, findings, conclusions, or recommendations expressed in this article do not necessarily represent those of the National Endowment for the Humanities.

CONFLICTS OF INTEREST

The author declares no conflicts of interest.

ENDNOTES

1. See, for instance, Elaine Tyler May, *America and the Pill: A History of Promise, Peril, and Liberation* (New York, NY: Basic Books, 2011); Elizabeth Siegel Watkins, *On the Pill: A Social History of Oral Contraceptives, 1950–1970* (Baltimore, MD: Johns Hopkins University Press, 2001). The history of US birth control more generally and especially before the pill is a vast field explored extensively in Ellen Chesler, *Woman of Valor: Margaret Sanger and the Birth Control Movement in America* (New York, NY: Simon & Schuster, 2007); Linda Gordon, *The Moral Property of Women: A History of Birth Control Politics in America* (Urbana, IL: University of Illinois Press, 2007); Carole R. McCann, *Birth-Control Politics in the United States, 1916–1945* (Ithaca, NY: Cornell University Press, 1999); and James Reed, *From Private Vice to Public Virtue: The Birth Control Movement and American Society Since 1830* (New York, NY: Basic Books, 1978).
2. Cathy Moran Hajo, *Birth Control on Main Street: Organizing Clinics in the United States, 1916–1939* (Urbana, IL: University of Illinois Press, 2010); Melissa R. Klapper, *Ballots, Babies, and Banners of Peace* (New York, NY: New York University Press, 2013). By 1937, there were approximately 320 functioning birth control clinics in the United States: "A New Day Dawns for Birth Control" (New York, NY: National Committee Federal Legislation for Birth Control, 1937).
3. Hannah M. Stone, "Therapeutic Contraception," *Medical Journal and Record* (March 1928): 9–17. After this initial publication, US medical journals such as the *American Journal of Public Health* and the *Journal of the American Medical Association* began publishing articles on contraception with increasing regularity.
4. *People v. Sanger*, 222 NY 192 (1918).
5. Margaret Sanger, "Hannah M. Stone—In Memoriam," *Human Fertility* 6, no. 4 (August 1941): 109.
6. See, for instance, Anu Manchikanti Gomez, Liza Fuentes, and Amy Allina, "Women or LARC First? Reproductive Autonomy and the Promotion of Long-Acting Reversible Contraceptive Methods," *Perspectives on Sexual and Reproductive Health* 46, no. 3 (2014): 171–175; Michelle H. Moniz et al., "Inpatient Postpartum Long-Acting Reversible Contraception: Care That Promotes Reproductive Justice," *Obstetrics and Gynecology* 130, no. 4 (2017): 783–787.
7. Act of the Suppression of Trade in, and Circulation of, Obscene Literature and Articles of Immoral Use, Ch 258, 17 Stat 596-600 (1873).
8. *People v. Sanger*.
9. Hajo, *Birth Control on Main Street*, 6.
10. *United States v. One Package*, 86 F 2nd 737 (1936).
11. *Griswold v. Connecticut*, 381 US 479 (1965); *Eisenstadt v. Baird*, 405 US 438 (1972); and *Carey v. Population Services International*, 431 US 678 (1977).
12. Sanger, "Hannah M. Stone—In Memoriam," 109.
13. Robert L. Dickinson, "Hannah M. Stone—In Memoriam," *Human Fertility* 6, no. 4 (August 1941): 111.
14. Chesler, *Woman of Valor*, 278–279.
15. Gregory Stragnell to Hannah Mayer Stone, 15 December 1925, box 36, folder 4, Margaret Sanger Papers, Sophia Smith Collection of Women's History, Smith College.
16. Irving H. Jurow to Hannah M. Stone, 12 January 1937, box 36, folder 5, Margaret Sanger Papers, Sophia Smith Collection of Women's History, Smith College.
17. Gordon, *The Moral Property of Women*, 181–182.
18. Robert L. Dickinson, "Open Forum: Birth Control," *Medical Journal and Record* (March 1928): 7.
19. Clinic patients were required to be married and not pregnant. Services were offered for free to those who could not afford to pay, and members of immigrant communities were recruited with informational materials translated into multiple languages. A small percentage of Black women visited the clinic, many of whom commuted from Harlem: McCann, *Birth-Control Politics*.
20. Sanger, "Hannah M. Stone—In Memoriam," 109.
21. Janet Farrell Brodie, *Contraception and Abortion in 19th-Century America* (Ithaca, NY: Cornell University Press, 1994); Nicola Beisel, *Imperiled Innocents: Anthony Comstock and Family Reproduction in Victorian America* (Princeton, NJ: Princeton University Press, 1997).
22. Ellen S. More, *The Transformation of American Sex Education: Mary Calderone and the Fight for Sexual Health* (New York, NY: New York University Press, 2022).
23. Stone, "Therapeutic Contraception," 12.
24. Stone, "Therapeutic Contraception," 11.
25. Stone, "Therapeutic Contraception," 13.
26. Stone, "Therapeutic Contraception," 17.
27. Hannah M. Stone to Doctor, 27 June 1933, box 36, folder 4, Margaret Sanger Papers, Sophia Smith Collection of Women's History, Smith College.
28. Ibid.
29. Hannah M. Stone to Lydia Allen DeVilbiss, 25 September 1935, box 36, folder 4, Margaret Sanger Papers, Sophia Smith Collection of Women's History, Smith College.
30. Hannah M. Stone to birth control organizations in the United States, 2 May 1938, box 36, folder 5, Margaret Sanger Papers, Sophia Smith Collection of Women's History, Smith College.
31. Hannah M. Stone to Lydia Allen DeVilbiss, 1 June 1935, box 36, folder 4, Margaret Sanger Papers, Sophia Smith Collection of Women's History, Smith College.
32. Hannah M. Stone to Robert L. Dickinson, 22 March 1938, box 36, folder 5, Margaret Sanger Papers, Sophia Smith Collection of Women's History, Smith College.
33. Woman's Activities to Hannah Stone, 8 March 1932, box 12, folder 28, Abraham Stone Papers, Francis A. Countway Library of Medicine, Harvard University.
34. Hannah M. Stone to Frieda L. Greenson, 4 February 1937, box 36, folder 5, Margaret Sanger Papers, Sophia Smith Collection of Women's History, Smith College.
35. Hannah M. Stone to Lily Sendra, 12 September 1938, box 36, folder 5, Margaret Sanger Papers, Sophia Smith Collection of Women's History, Smith College.
36. Nikita M. Malcolm et al., "Using Evidence to Expand Contraceptive Access," *American Journal of Public Health* 112, no. S5 (June 2022): S470–S472.

37. Loretta J. Ross, "Reproductive Justice as Intersectional Feminist Activism," *Souls* 19, no. 3 (2017): 286–314; Loretta Ross and Rickie Solinger, *Reproductive Justice: An Introduction* (Berkeley, CA: University of California Press, 2017).

38. Dorothy Roberts, *Killing the Black Body: Race, Reproduction, and the Meaning of Liberty* (New York, NY: Pantheon Press, 1997); Harriet A. Washington, *Medical Apartheid: The Dark History of Medical Experimentation on Black Americans From Colonial Times to the Present* (New York, NY: Broadway Books, 2006).

Minor Consent Laws for Sexually Transmitted Infection and Human Immunodeficiency Virus Services in the United States: A Comprehensive, Longitudinal Survey of US State Laws

Kimberly M. Nelson, PhD, MPH, Alexandra Skinner, MPH, Claire D. Stout, BA, Will Raderman, MSc, Emily Unger, PhD, Julia Raifman, ScD, SM, Madina Agénor, ScD, MPH, Michele L. Ybarra, PhD, MPH, Shira I. Dunsiger, PhD, S. Bryn Austin, ScD, SM, and Kristen Underhill, DPhil, JD

See also Hill, p. 350.

Objectives. To assess changes in minor consent laws for sexually transmitted infection (STI) and HIV testing, treatment, and prevention services in all 50 US states and the District of Columbia from 1900 to 2021.

Methods. We coded laws into minor consent for (1) health care generally; (2) STI testing, treatment, and prevention; (3) HIV testing, treatment, and prevention; and (4) pre- or postexposure prophylaxis for HIV prevention. We also coded confidentiality protections and required conditions (e.g., threshold clinician judgments).

Results. The largest increase in states allowing minors to consent to STI services occurred during the 1960s and 1970s. By 2021, minors could consent independently to STI and HIV testing and treatment in all 50 states plus DC, STI prevention services in 32 jurisdictions, and HIV prevention services in 33 jurisdictions. Confidentiality protections for minors are rare. Prerequisites are common.

Conclusions. Although the number of states allowing minors to consent independently to STI and HIV services has increased considerably, these laws have substantial limitations, including high complexity, prerequisites requiring clinician judgments, and neglect of confidentiality concerns. (*Am J Public Health.* 2023;113(4):397–407. https://doi.org/10.2105/AJPH.2022.307199)

AJPH April 2023, Vol 113, No. 4

Adolescents in the United States are significantly burdened by sexually transmitted infections (STIs), including HIV.[1,2] Sexual, gender, and racial/ethnic minority adolescents are disproportionately affected.[1,2] Despite elevated risk of STI and HIV transmission and clinical recommendations for routine screening and access to prevention services,[3,4] STI and HIV testing rates and use of preventive care, including pre- and postexposure prophylaxis (PrEP and PEP, respectively), are low among adolescents who are having sex.[5,6] There are also pronounced inequities in STI and HIV service use by sexual orientation, gender, and race/ethnicity.[5,6]

Guardian consent requirements are a significant barrier to care for minors who are unable or unwilling to involve their guardian when they are seeking STI or HIV services.[7–9] Minors seeking STI or HIV services may need to disclose information about their sexual activity, sexual orientation, or gender identity to their clinician and guardian. These disclosures can be difficult, risky, or impossible for adolescents whose guardians may react with discipline, rejection, or abuse, or for adolescents who are unstably housed, not living with their guardian, institutionalized, or in foster care.[7–9] To address this obstacle, states have enacted statutes granting minors legal capacity to consent to STI and HIV services without their guardians' consent. These statutes benefit both minors and clinicians; they reduce minors' barriers to STI and HIV care, and they enable clinicians to provide services without risking legal repercussions because of their patients' age. Since 1970, US minors have also had the capacity to consent independently to family planning services, including STI and HIV services, delivered through federal Title X program grants.[10] Although Title X programs are helpful, there are substantial limitations to adolescent uptake,[11–13] and most minors receive care in clinicians' offices.[14] State statutes granting minors legal capacity to independently consent to STI and HIV services, therefore, remain critical.

Research on the impact of minor consent laws on the use of STI and HIV services among adolescents is limited.[15–18] One potential contributor to the lack of research in this area is the absence of rigorous, longitudinal data mapping the history of these laws and the complex conditions and confidentiality protections that are involved when minors independently seek care. Previous reviews of minor consent laws for STI and HIV services are cross-sectional, dated, and methodologically unclear, and they lack data on required conditions (e.g., threshold clinician judgments) and confidentiality requirements.[19–27]

This article extends and elaborates on existing reviews[19–27] by examining minor consent laws for STI and HIV services, including prerequisites and confidentiality protections, in all 50 states and the District of Columbia from 1900 to 2021. This longitudinal analysis of state law will be useful for legal, policy, and public health researchers who can capitalize on the natural experiments created by differences in the laws over time and between states. Furthermore, the detailed accounting of the current law can inform clinical practice and identify areas where additional legal protections are necessary. The goal of this work is to facilitate research, practice, and policies that will reduce barriers to STI and HIV care for adolescents and promote sexual health equity nationwide.

METHODS

Using best practices for creating longitudinal data sets of state health laws,[28] our team followed a replicable process of identifying, double coding, reconciling, and analyzing relevant laws. The objective was to generate a legal survey of state statutes (enacted by legislatures), state regulations (enacted by state agencies), and state and federal case law (judges' decisions) regulating the legal capacity of minors in each state and DC to consent to STI and HIV testing, treatment, and prevention services without guardian permission. We divided laws into 4 categories: (1) consent to health care generally; (2) consent to STI testing, treatment, or prevention; (3) consent to HIV testing, treatment, or prevention; and (4) consent to PrEP or PEP for HIV prevention. We also surveyed confidentiality protections that may allow or require clinicians to avoid disclosing health care information to guardians, as well as laws that protect against health care payor communications (e.g., explanation of benefits [EOB]) disclosure to guardians. Because we defined "minors" as people below a state's legal age of majority, we coded state laws on majority age. We also identified specific conditions that some states require before granting minors legal capacity to consent to care.

Although Congress could enact a federal statute on minors' capacity to access health care, they have not done so. With the exception of care delivered in Title X grantee programs, states decide minors' capacity to consent to care. As such, our data set summarizes state law.

We generated a list of legal variables and coding schemes, defining each variable with a preset list of responses. We revised the coding schemes after coding 5 preliminary states. Four legal research assistants conducted initial coding during June through December 2020 by systematically searching, collecting, and coding state legislation, regulations, and judicial decisions in Westlaw for each jurisdiction. They used separate search strings for laws regulating minor consent to general health care (<[minor! adolesc! child! age!]/p ["medical care" "health" "healthcare" doctor! physician! provider! treat! prevent! diagnos!] >) and laws regulating minor consent to HIV and STI care (<[minor! adolesc! child! age!]/p [HIV STI STD sexual! venereal immunodeficien!] >). Because our focus was on STI and HIV care, we excluded laws focusing exclusively on reproductive health care and family planning, including contraception and abortion. Searches for cases included both state and federal cases applicable in each jurisdiction.

Where we identified a relevant state law, we tracked the legal rule backward through all available past versions, examining any changes since its enactment. We recorded any changes that affected our variables of interest. We were occasionally unable to obtain versions of legislation from specific past years. In these situations, we used all available contextual information to identify possible changes at the missing time point (e.g., legislative history, legislative findings, case law, editors' comments), and if we could not identify a change, we assumed that no relevant changes were made. Because a majority of amendments were nonsubstantive for our variables of interest, this was a conservative assumption. All relevant citations were Shepardized, a process of tracking citations to examine any cases or legislative changes that may have affected the validity or application of the law.

We abstracted data from legal source material into an Excel spreadsheet for each state, noting all relevant amendments and their years. All data were redundantly collected and coded by 2 independent research assistants who reconciled discrepancies by discussion and referral to the legal expert on our team (K. U). We compared findings to existing cross-sectional surveys to ensure completeness and reviewed all findings to identify coding errors.

After initial coding was complete, 2 independent researchers (C. S. and W. R.), analyzed each state to prepare a master set of rules. Data were cleaned and updated in a collaborative process between the team's legal and public health researchers in October 2021, which involved applying this master set of rules, checking the most up-to-date laws, and revising data to include any updates since initial coding.

For each type of care, we identified the youngest age at which mentally competent minors have capacity to consent independently. Where multiple laws provided capacity to consent to the same type of care, we coded the youngest age at which the minor has capacity to consent both with conditions and without conditions. Mental capacity to consent is already a prerequisite to providing informed consent in every state. As such, we did not code redundant conditions that specified that minors would need mental capacity.

Furthermore, although some analyses and popular press articles have labeled certain minor consent laws as being PrEP-specific,[27,29] these statutes are worded in terms of HIV prevention generally; thus, we did not separate PrEP from HIV prevention in our results. States adopted minor consent for testing and treatment concurrently; in each state, the youngest age of allowable consent to testing (for STI or HIV) was the same as that for treatment. We therefore present STI and HIV testing and treatment jointly in our results. Legal citations are available in Table A (available as a supplement to the online version of this article at https://ajph.org). State-specific data on age of majority and youngest age of legal capacity of mentally competent minors to consent to STI and HIV care from 1900 to 2021 are available in Tables B and C (available as supplements to the online version of this article at https://ajph.org). Additional details about procedures, assumptions, and definitions have been published previously.[30]

RESULTS

The number of states allowing minors to consent independently to STI and HIV services has increased considerably in the past century.

1900–1959

Between 1900 and 1959, minors were allowed to consent independently to general care in 1 state, STI testing and treatment in 9 states, and STI prevention services in 1 state (Figure 1). In Massachusetts, minors were able to consent independently to STI testing and treatment only if the services were provided in a public clinic. No other states required conditions. Only 2 states had laws that specified confidentiality protections for minors (Table 1), both of which stated that it was a clinician's discretion whether they kept the services confidential from guardians.

1960–1979

During the 1960s and 1970s, there was a substantial increase in the number of states that allowed minors to consent independently to general care (14 jurisdictions), STI testing and treatment (41 jurisdictions), and STI-prevention services (21 jurisdictions; Figure 1). However, multiple states had conditions that must be met. Among the most common conditions were 2 prerequisites: (1) in the clinician's judgment, delaying care would substantially increase the risk to the minor's life or health or (2) the patient believes themselves to be afflicted with a relevant illness or disease. Additional conditions are captured in Table B.

By 1979, among the 41 jurisdictions that allowed minors to consent independently to STI testing and treatment, 17 specified confidentiality protections for minors who access these services (Table 1). One state had distinct levels of confidentiality protections for STI testing versus treatment; in South Dakota, confidentiality protections applied for minors seeking STI treatment (according to the clinician's discretion), but not for STI testing. Among the 21 jurisdictions that allowed minors to consent independently to STI prevention services during this period, 11 specified confidentiality protections for minors who access these services (Table 1).

1980–1999

Steady growth in the number of states allowing minors to consent independently

AJPH April 2023, Vol 113, No. 4

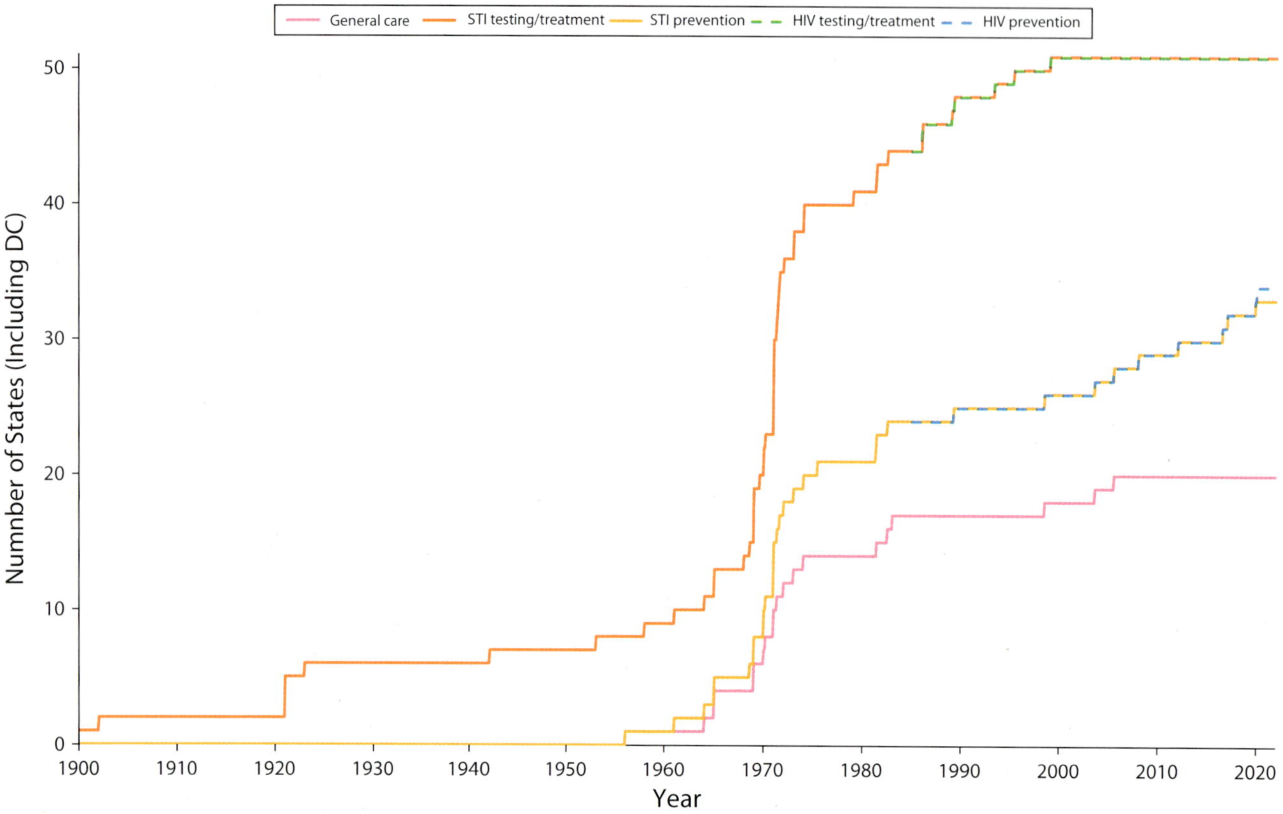

FIGURE 1— Number of US States That Granted Minors Legal Capacity to Consent to Health Care: 1900–2021

Note. STI = sexually transmitted infection. Minor consent laws for HIV testing, treatment, and HIV prevention are depicted beginning in 1985, the year in which the first HIV antibody test became available.[31]

to general care and STI services continued during the 1980s and 1990s. Minors also gained the ability to consent to HIV testing, treatment, and prevention services in some states. By December 1999, minors were able to consent independently to general care in 17 jurisdictions, STI testing and treatment in all 50 states plus DC, and STI prevention services in 25 jurisdictions (Figure 1). Furthermore, minors could independently consent to HIV testing and treatment in all 50 states plus DC and to HIV prevention services in 25 jurisdictions (Figure 1). Many states continued existing conditions or added additional prerequisites, as captured in Tables B and C.

Among the 51 jurisdictions that allowed minors to consent independently to STI testing and treatment, 24 specified confidentiality protections for minors who access these services (Table 1). South Dakota's protections remained distinct for STI testing versus treatment. Among the 25 jurisdictions that allowed minors to consent independently to STI-prevention services, 13 specified confidentiality protections (Table 1). Among the 51 jurisdictions that allowed minors to consent independently to HIV testing and treatment, 23 specified confidentiality protections (Table 2). One state had distinct levels of confidentiality protections for HIV testing versus treatment; in Delaware, there were confidentiality protections for minors seeking HIV testing (according to the clinician's discretion), but none for HIV treatment. Among the 25 jurisdictions that allowed minors to consent independently to HIV-prevention services, 13 specified confidentiality protections for minors who access these services (Table 2). Lastly, as of 1986, when a minor receives any health care without guardian consent in Florida, their health care payor EOB form and other communications (i.e., billing, online claims records) are protected against disclosure to guardians (Table 3).

2000–2021

From 2000 through 2021, the number of states allowing minors to consent to STI- and HIV-prevention services continued to increase. As of December 2021, minors can independently consent to general care in 20 states, STI and HIV testing and treatment in all

TABLE 1— State-Level Confidentiality Protections for Minors' Sexually Transmitted Infection Care Information: United States, 1900–2021

State	Years	STI Testing	STI Treatment	STI Prevention
Alabama[a]	1900–1970	—	—	—
	1971–2021	N	N	N
Alaska	1900–1973	—	—	—
	1974–2021	N	N	—
Arizona	1900–1970	—	—	—
	1971–2021	N	N	—
Arkansas	1900–1968	—	—	—
	1969–1972	N	N	—
	1973–2021	N	N	N
California	1900–1967	—	—	—
	1968–2011	N	N	—
	2012–2021	N	N	N
Colorado	1900–1920	—	—	—
	1921–2015	N	N	—
	2016–2021	MC[b]	MC[b]	MC[b]
Connecticut	1900–1957	—	—	—
	1958–1995	N	N	—
	1996–2021	MC	MC	—
Delaware	1900–1963	—	—	—
	1964–2011	N	N	N
	2012–2021	CD	CD	CD
District of Columbia	1900–1973	—	—	—
	1974–2021	CD	CD	CD
Florida	1900–1985	—	—	—
	1986–2021	MC	MC	—
Georgia	1900–1970	—	—	—
	1971–2021	N	N	—
Hawaii	1900–1978	—	—	—
	1979–2021	N	N	—
Idaho	1900–1970	—	—	—
	1971–2004	N	N	—
	2005–2021	N	N	N
Illinois	1900–1960	N	N	N
	1961–2021	MC	MC	MC
Indiana	1900–1992	—	—	—
	1993–2021	N	N	—
Iowa	1900–1998	—	—	—
	1999–2007	N	N	—
	2008–2021	N	N	N
Kansas	1900–1968	—	—	—
	1969–2021	N	N	N
Kentucky	1900–1969	—	—	—
	1970–2021	CD	CD	N

Continued

50 states plus DC, STI-prevention services in 32 jurisdictions, and HIV-prevention services in 33 jurisdictions (Figure 1). Prerequisites continue to be common, as captured in Tables B and C.

Confidentiality protections changed minimally during this period. Among the 51 jurisdictions that allowed minors to consent independently to STI testing and treatment, 27 specified confidentiality protections for minors who access these services (Table 1). Among the 32 jurisdictions that allowed minors to consent independently to STI-prevention services, 17 specified confidentiality protections (Table 1). Among the 51 jurisdictions that allowed minors to consent independently to HIV testing and treatment, 29 specified confidentiality protections (Table 2). Among the 33 jurisdictions that allowed minors to consent independently to HIV-prevention services, 18 specified confidentiality protections (Table 2).

Lastly, additional states adopted payor-related protection provisions (Table 3). Specifically, Colorado, New York, and Washington joined Florida in protecting health care payor EOBs against disclosure to guardians when a minor receives any health care without guardian consent. Similarly, Delaware, New York, and Washington joined Florida in protecting other communications from the health care payor (i.e., billing, online claims records) against disclosure to guardians when a minor receives any health care without guardian consent.

DISCUSSION

Adolescents in the United States are disproportionately affected by STIs and HIV and require access to testing, treatment, and prevention services.[1,2] Laws that give minors capacity to consent to care are important for minors who are

AJPH April 2023, Vol 113, No. 4

TABLE 1— Continued

State	Years	STI Testing	STI Treatment	STI Prevention
Louisiana	1900–1969	—	—	—
	1970–2021	CD	CD	CD
Maine	1900–1970	—	—	—
	1971–2018	CD	CD	—
	2019–2021	CD	CD	CD
Maryland	1900–1981	—	—	—
	1982–2021	CD	CD	CD
Massachusetts	1900–1974	N	N	—
	1975–2021	MC[c]	MC[c]	—
Michigan	1900–1988	—	—	—
	1989–2021	CD	CD	CD
Minnesota	1900–1970	—	—	—
	1971–2021	MC[d]	MC[d]	MC[d]
Mississippi[a]	1900–1941	—	—	—
	1942–1997	CD	CD	—
	1998–2021	CD	CD	N
Missouri	1900–1970	—	—	—
	1971–2021	MC[e]	MC[e]	MC[e]
Montana	1900–1968	—	—	—
	1969–2021	N	N	N
Nebraska[a]	1900–1971	—	—	—
	1972–2021	CD	CD	CD
Nevada	1900–1964	—	—	—
	1965–2021	MC	MC	MC
New Hampshire	1900–1985	—	—	—
	1986–2021	CD	CD	—
New Jersey	1900–1967	—	—	—
	1968–2021	CD	CD	CD
New Mexico	1900–1972	—	—	—
	1973–2021	N	N	—
New York	1900–1952	—	—	—
	1953–2015	N	N	—
	2016–2021	MC	MC	MC
North Carolina	1900–1964	—	—	—
	1965–1976	N	N	N
	1977–2021	MC[f]	MC[f]	MC[f]
North Dakota	1900–1970	—	—	—
	1971–2021	N	N	N
Ohio	1900–1970	—	—	—
	1971–2021	N	N	—
Oklahoma	1900–1970	—	—	—
	1971–1974	N	N	—
	1975–2021	MC[e]	MC[e]	MC[e]
Oregon	1900–1968	—	—	—
	1969–1970	N	N	—
	1971–2021	N	N	CD

Continued

unable or unwilling to involve guardians when they are seeking STI and HIV services.[7–9] These laws may be especially critical for addressing the STI and HIV inequities experienced by marginalized youths.[9]

Many minor consent statutes on STI testing and treatment date back to the earliest years of the 20th century and are written with reference to "venereal disease." Minor consent statutes in this era reflect Progressive concerns about STIs among young people and members of the armed forces, as well as Reformer beliefs that STIs were an acute threat to childbearing and marriage.[32] States in this era enacted minor consent laws that enabled STI testing before marriage or enlistment for people who married or registered for the military before the age of majority (often age 21).

The number of states allowing minors to consent independently to STI services increased slowly until the late 1960s and early 1970s, when there was a dramatic increase in states adopting these statutes. Social changes (e.g., civil rights activism, the sexual revolution), sexual health advances (e.g., the introduction of birth control pills and intrauterine devices, the inception of Title X grants), legal developments (e.g., nondiscrimination laws), and an increased understanding of minors' capacity all likely contributed to the evolution of minor consent statutes during this time.[33] These decades also saw landmark court decisions identifying individual due process rights to access contraception (e.g., *Eisenstadt v Baird*) and abortion (e.g., *Roe v Wade*). The 1960s and 1970s also drew attention to children as "rights-bearing persons," and children's rights advocates emphasized that minors had needs and interests that were separate from those of

TABLE 1— Continued

State	Years	STI Testing	STI Treatment	STI Prevention
Pennsylvania[a]	1900–1969	—	—	—
	1970–2021	N	N	N
Rhode Island	1900–1922	—	—	—
	1923–1955	N	N	—
	1956–2021	N	N	N
South Carolina	1900–1980	—	—	—
	1981–2021	N	N	N
South Dakota	1900–1970	—	—	—
	1971–2021	N	CD	N
Tennessee	1900–1920	—	—	—
	1921–2002	CD	CD	—
	2003–2021	CD	CD	N
Texas	1900–1994	—	—	—
	1995–2021	CD	CD	—
Utah	1900–1980	—	—	—
	1981–2021	N	N	N
Vermont	1900–1970	—	—	—
	1971–2021	N	N	—
Virginia	1900–1988	—	—	—
	1989–1998	N	N	—
	1999–2021	MC	MC	—
Washington	1900–1968	—	—	—
	1969–2021	N	N	—
West Virginia	1900–1920	—	—	—
	1921–2021	CD	CD	—
Wisconsin	1900–1916	—	—	—
	1917–2021	N	N	—
Wyoming	1900–1972	—	—	—
	1973–2021	MC	MC	—

Note. CD = clinician discretion; MC = mandatory confidentiality; N = no confidentiality protections; STI = sexually transmitted infection. A dash (—) indicates that minors do not have the legal capacity to consent to that service.

[a]Age of majority is > 18 y.
[b]Clinician discretion if minor is younger than 14 years.
[c]Clinician must disclose minor health information to parent or guardian if the condition of said minor is so serious that life or limb is endangered.
[d]Clinician discretion if failure to inform parent or guardian would seriously jeopardize the health of the minor patient.
[e]Clinician discretion if test is positive.
[f]Clinician discretion if contacted by parent or guardian.

their guardians and the state.[34] Many courts, including the Supreme Court (e.g., *Bellotti v Baird*), made decisions that recognized an independent legal and developmental status for minors during this time.

Adoption of minor consent statutes for STI services continued to slowly increase through 1999, by which time every jurisdiction allowed minors to consent independently to STI testing and treatment. When HIV testing became widely available in 1985,[31] many states already had sufficiently expansive STI testing and treatment minor consent laws for them to apply to HIV services as well. Other states passed new HIV-specific laws throughout the 1980s and 1990s to accommodate HIV testing and treatment. These laws reflected keen attention to HIV as a health risk for adolescents during the peak of the national HIV epidemic (i.e., 1981–1996) and before the widespread availability of highly active antiretroviral therapy.

Since 2000, laws have increasingly focused on facilitating minors' access to biomedical STI and HIV prevention (e.g., human papillomavirus vaccination, PrEP, PEP). Because STI and HIV prevention in earlier eras was mostly limited to over-the-counter barrier methods (e.g., condoms), many earlier laws specifically named access to testing and treatment but not prevention. Generic laws allowing minors to consent to STI and HIV "care" or "services" are broad enough to encompass prevention, and some states have amended their laws to include prevention explicitly. But, in states without these features, capacity to consent to STI and HIV prevention still depends on whether there is a right to consent to general medical care that includes preventive care. Without these options, the legal age of majority is the earliest that young people can independently consent to STI and HIV prevention.

Critically, across all years, most states have neglected or only cursorily addressed confidentiality obligations for clinicians who deliver care to independently consenting minors. In states where there are no explicit laws protecting the confidentiality of minors' STI or HIV services, default rules under the Health Insurance Portability and

TABLE 2— State-Level Confidentiality Protections for Minors' HIV Care Information: United States, 1985–2021

State	Years	HIV Testing	HIV Treatment	HIV Prevention
Alabama[a]	1985–2021	N	N	N
Alaska	1985–2021	N	N	—
Arizona	1985–2021	N	N	—
Arkansas	1985–2021	N	N	N
California	1985–2011	N	N	—
	2012–2021	N	N	N
Colorado	1985–2015	N	N	—
	2016–2021	MC[b]	MC[b]	MC[b]
Connecticut	1985–2018	MC	MC	—
	2019–2021	MC	MC	MC
Delaware	1985–1987	N	N	N
	1988–2011	CD	N	N
	2012–2021	CD	CD	CD
District of Columbia	1985–2021	CD	CD	CD
Florida	1985–2013	N	MC	—
	2014–2021	MC	MC	—
Georgia	1985–2021	N	N	—
Hawaii	1985–2021	N	N	—
Idaho	1985–2004	N	N	—
	2005–2021	N	N	N
Illinois	1985–2021	MC	MC	MC
Indiana	1985–1992	—	—	—
	1993–2021	N	N	—
Iowa	1985–1998	—	—	—
	1999–2007	N	N	—
	2008–2021	N	N	N
Kansas	1985–2021	N	N	N
Kentucky	1985–2021	CD	CD	N
Louisiana	1985–2021	CD	CD	CD
Maine	1985–2018	CD	CD	—
	2019–2021	CD	CD	CD
Maryland	1985–2021	CD	CD	CD
Massachusetts	1985–2021	MC[c]	MC[c]	—
Michigan	1985–1988	—	—	—
	1989–2021	CD	CD	CD
Minnesota	1985–2021	MC[d]	MC[d]	MC[c]
Mississippi[a]	1985–1997	CD	CD	—
	1998–2021	CD	CD	N
Missouri	1985–2021	CD	MC[e]	MC[e]
Montana	1985–2021	N	N	N
Nebraska[a]	1985–2021	CD	CD	CD
Nevada	1985–2021	MC	MC	MC
New Hampshire	1985–1985	—	—	—
	1986–2021	CD	CD	—

Continued

Accountability Act allow guardians to access their children's medical records. The Act also allows clinicians to exercise discretion over disclosures "to the extent allowed by law" when minors consent independently to care and where states have no law on the subject. Where states have their own laws on confidentiality, these take priority.

Among states that have addressed confidentiality, the most common rule is to allow clinicians to exercise discretion over which information they disclose to guardians. More rarely, some states require that clinicians keep information about care confidential, with some exceptions for permissible or required disclosures (e.g., when the clinician believes that nondisclosure would jeopardize the health of the minor patient). For minors who may face rejection or abuse, the capacity to consent to their own care is incomplete and fraught if their clinicians can, or must, disclose their information to guardians.

Very few states address insurance billing and claims processes that may inadvertently break confidentiality. Only a handful of states have acted to protect EOBs and other records against disclosure to guardians. Because the majority of adolescents are covered by their guardians' insurance,[35] inadvertent disclosure through payment processes is a substantial barrier to care for adolescents and could be dangerous for youths who face rejection or abuse if receipt of services is disclosed. It is critical that states address these potential loopholes to confidentiality. At the point of care, clinicians should help minors understand their payment options (e.g., insurance, paying out of pocket, locating free services) and their implications for maintaining confidentiality.

TABLE 2— Continued

State	Years	HIV Testing	HIV Treatment	HIV Prevention
New Jersey	1985–2021	CD	CD	CD
New Mexico	1985–2021	N	N	—
New York	1985–2015	N	N	—
	2016	MC	MC	—
	2017–2021	MC	MC	MC
North Carolina	1985–2021	MC[f]	MC[f]	MC[f]
North Dakota	1985–2021	N	N	N
Ohio	1985–2021	N	N	—
Oklahoma	1985–2021	MC[e]	MC[e]	MC[e]
Oregon	1985–2021	N	N	CD
Pennsylvania[a]	1985–2021	N	N	N
Rhode Island	1985–2021	N	N	N
South Carolina	1985–2021	N	N	N
South Dakota	1985–2021	N	CD	N
Tennessee	1985–2002	CD	CD	—
	2003–2021	CD	CD	N
Texas	1985–1994	—	—	—
	1995–2021	CD	CD	—
Utah	1985–2008	N	N	N
	2009–2021	MC	N	N
Vermont	1985–2021	N	N	—
Virginia	1985–1988	—	—	—
	1989–1998	N	N	—
	1999–2021	MC	MC	—
Washington	1985–2019	N	N	—
	2020–2021	N	N	N
West Virginia	1985–2021	CD	CD	—
Wisconsin	1985–2021	MC	N	—
Wyoming	1985–2021	MC	MC	—

Note. CD = clinician discretion; MC = mandatory confidentiality; N = no confidentiality protections. A dash (—) indicates that minors do not have the legal capacity to consent to that service.

[a]Age of majority is > 18 y.
[b]Clinician discretion if minor is younger than 14 years.
[c]Clinician must disclose minor health information to parent or guardian if the condition of said minor is so serious that life or limb is endangered.
[d]Clinician discretion if failure to inform parent or guardian would seriously jeopardize the health of the minor patient.
[e]Clinician discretion if test is positive.
[f]Clinician discretion if contacted by parent or guardian.

Strengths and Limitations

Our study has many strengths, including our longitudinal approach to tracking laws from their inception, our canvassing of not only state statutes but also judicial opinions and regulations, our systematic approach to redundant coding and reconciliation, and our simultaneous application of multiple sets of laws that affect minors' capacity to consent to STI and HIV testing, treatment, and prevention services. Furthermore, our study provides critical information about potential conditions and confidentiality protections for adolescents who are independently seeking STI and HIV services in each state. This information is necessary to gain a full understanding of what is required for adolescents to independently obtain these services and maintain their confidentiality.

Our study also has limitations. We did not assess municipal law, and cities within individual states may have differing rules. We also did not assess the full scope of minor consent statutes related to sexual health (e.g., contraception, abortion) but, rather, focused only on laws pertinent to STI and HIV care. Laws that did not mention STIs or HIV (e.g., laws that only included "family planning") were not retrieved by our search. As mental capacity to consent is already a prerequisite to providing informed consent in every state, our findings do not apply to minors who lack mental competence. In addition, our search was not optimized to identify laws that had been long discontinued, for which an updated or repealed version would have been unavailable at the time of our initial Westlaw queries. We also acknowledge that minors who access STI and HIV care through Title X grantee programs have capacity to consent independently regardless of state law.

Public Health Implications

Increasing STI and HIV testing, treatment, and prevention service use is key to decreasing STI and HIV rates among adolescents in the United States. Minor consent laws were enacted for the purpose of expanding access to care. Although the number of states allowing minors to consent independently to STI and HIV services has increased

TABLE 3— State-Level Laws Protecting Minors' Health Care Payor Information From Disclosure to Guardians: United States, 1900–2021

State	Years	Explanation of Benefits	Other Communications From Health Care Payor
Colorado	2018–2021	Y	N
Delaware	2012–2021	N	Y
Florida	1986–2021	Y	Y
New York	2016–2021	Y	Y
Washington	2001–2021	Y	Y

Note. N = no protections against disclosure to guardians; Y = protected against disclosure to guardians when a minor receives any health care without guardian consent. Jurisdictions not included in this table have no history of nor current protections of minors' health care payor information against disclosure to guardians.

considerably over the past century, these laws have substantial limitations, including being complex, relying on clinician judgments, and leaving significant confidentiality concerns unaddressed. Understanding the history, intricate structure, and limitations of these laws is essential to assess their impacts on access, to inform clinical practice, to identify areas where additional legal protections are necessary, and, ultimately, to promote sexual health equity and access to care for US adolescents. AJPH

ABOUT THE AUTHORS

Kimberly M. Nelson and Claire D. Stout are with the Department of Community Health Sciences, Boston University School of Public Health, Boston, MA. Alexandra Skinner, Will Raderman, and Julia Raifman are with the Department of Health Law, Policy, and Management, Boston University School of Public Health. Emily Unger and S. Bryn Austin are with the Department of Social and Behavioral Sciences, Harvard T. H. Chan School of Public Health, Boston. Madina Agénor and Shira I. Dunsiger are with the Department of Behavioral and Social Sciences, Brown University School of Public Health, Providence, RI. Michele L. Ybarra is with the Center for Innovative Public Health Research, San Clemente, CA. Kristen Underhill is with Cornell Law School, Ithaca, NY.

CORRESPONDENCE

Correspondence should be sent to Kimberly Nelson, PhD, MPH, Boston University School of Public Health, 801 Massachusetts Ave, 4th Floor, Boston, MA 02118 (e-mail: knel@bu.edu). Reprints can be ordered at https://ajph.org by clicking the "Reprints" link.

PUBLICATION INFORMATION

Full Citation: Nelson KM, Skinner A, Stout CD, et al. Minor consent laws for sexually transmitted infection and human immunodeficiency virus services in the United States: a comprehensive, longitudinal survey of US state laws. *Am J Public Health*. 2023;113(4):397–407.

Acceptance Date: December 2, 2022.

DOI: https://doi.org/10.2105/AJPH.2022.307199

CONTRIBUTORS

All authors made substantial contributions to this article. K. Nelson and K. Underhill conceptualized the study. K. Nelson acquired the funding. K. Underhill led the legal coding, cleaning, and updating process. C. Stout and W. Raderman conducted data cleaning and updating. K. Underhill in collaboration with E. Unger and A. Skinner finalized the data set. K. Nelson, K. Underhill, and A. Skinner wrote the initial article draft. J. Raifman, M. Agénor, M. Ybarra, S. Dunsiger, and S. B. Austin provided critical feedback throughout the development of the data set. All authors reviewed and edited the article.

ACKNOWLEDGMENTS

This work is supported by the National Institute of Mental Health (R01MH119892; PI: K. M. N.). S. B. Austin is supported by Maternal and Child Health Bureau, Health Resources and Services Administration grant T76-MC00001.

We would like to thank the Youth Advisory Board and the 4 law student research assistants who helped code the data.

Note. The content of this publication is solely the responsibility of the authors and does not represent the official views of the National Institutes of Health. The National Institutes of Health had no role in the design and conduct of the study; collection, management, analysis, and interpretation of the data; preparation, review, or approval of the article; or decision to submit the article for publication.

CONFLICTS OF INTEREST

The authors have no conflicts to report.

HUMAN PARTICIPANT PROTECTION

This study was exempted by the Boston University Medical Campus institutional review board.

REFERENCES

1. Centers for Disease Control and Prevention. Sexually transmitted disease surveillance, 2019. 2021. Available at: https://www.cdc.gov/std/statistics/2019/std-surveillance-2019.pdf. Accessed March 15, 2022.
2. Centers for Disease Control and Prevention. HIV Surveillance Report, 2019; Vol 32. 2021. Available at: http://www.cdc.gov/hiv/library/reports/hiv-surveillance.html. Accessed March 18, 2022.
3. Workowski KA, Bachmann LH, Chan PA, et al. Sexually transmitted infections treatment guidelines, 2021. *MMWR Recomm Rep.* 2021;70(4):1–187.
4. The Committee on Adolescence, Committee on Pediatric and Adolescent HIV, Section on Adolescent Health, Section on LGBT Health and Wellness. Adolescent sexual health AAP policy statements. American Academy of Pediatrics. 2022. Available at: http://www.aap.org/en/patient-care/adolescent-sexual-health/adolescent-sexual-health-aap-policy-statements. Accessed March 15, 2022.
5. Centers for Disease Control and Prevention. Youth Risk Behavior Survey data summary & trends report: 2009–2019. 2020. Available at: https://www.cdc.gov/healthyyouth/data/yrbs/pdf/YRBSDataSummaryTrendsReport2019-508.pdf. Accessed March 23, 2022.
6. Magnuson D, Hawkins T, Mera R. Adolescent use of Truvada (FTC/TDF) for HIV pre-exposure prophylaxis (PrEP) in the United States: (2012–2017). Presented at: 22nd International AIDS Conference; July 23–27, 2018; Amsterdam, the Netherlands. Available at: https://www.natap.org/2018/IAC/IAC_26.htm. Accessed March 15, 2022.
7. Cuffe KM, Newton-Levinson A, Gift TL, McFarlane M, Leichliter JS. Sexually transmitted infection testing among adolescents and young adults in the United States. *J Adolesc Health.* 2016;58(5):512–519. https://doi.org/10.1016/j.jadohealth.2016.01.002
8. Leichliter JS, Copen C, Dittus PJ. Confidentiality issues and use of sexually transmitted disease services among sexually experienced persons aged 15–25 years—United States, 2013–2015. *MMWR Morb Mortal Wkly Rep.* 2017;66(9):237–241. https://doi.org/10.15585/mmwr.mm6609a1
9. National Academies of Sciences, Engineering, and Medicine. *Sexually Transmitted Infections: Adopting a Sexual Health Paradigm.* Washington, DC: National Academies Press; 2021. https://doi.org/10.17226/25955
10. Congressional Research Service. Title X Family Planning Program. 2022. Available at: https://crsreports.congress.gov/product/pdf/IF/IF10051#:~:text=The%202021%20rule%20states%20

that,Title%20X%20family%20planning%20 services. Accessed November 9, 2022.

11. Krass P, Tam V, Min J, et al. Adolescent access to federally funded clinics providing confidential family planning following changes to Title X funding regulations. *JAMA Netw Open.* 2022;5(6): e2217488. https://doi.org/10.1001/jamanetwork open.2022.17488
12. US Department of Health and Human Services. Ensuring access to equitable, affordable, client-centered, quality family planning services. 86 FR 19812 (2021). Available at: https://www.federalregister.gov/documents/2021/04/15/2021-07762/ensuring-access-to-equitable-affordable-client-centered-quality-family-planning-services. Accessed November 9, 2022.
13. Wu JP, Van Sparrentak M, Waselewski M, DeJonckheere M, Remen R, Chang T. Youth opinions about Title X funding and policy in the United States: a mixed methods text message survey. *Contraception.* 2021;103(2):92–96. https://doi.org/10.1016/j.contraception.2020.10.008
14. Simon AE, Rossen LM, Schoendorf KC, Larson K, Olson LM. Location of usual source of care among children and adolescents in the United States, 1997–2013. *J Pediatr.* 2015;167(6): 1409–1414. https://doi.org/10.1016/j.jpeds.2015. 09.026
15. Nelson KM, Underhill K, Carey MP. Consent for HIV testing among adolescent sexual minority males: legal status, youth perceptions, and associations with actual testing and sexual risk behavior. *AIDS Behav.* 2020;24(2):373–378. https://doi.org/10.1007/s10461-019-02424-9
16. Pampati S, Liddon N, Dittus PJ, Adkins SH, Steiner RJ. Confidentiality matters but how do we improve implementation in adolescent sexual and reproductive health care? *J Adolesc Health.* 2019;65(3):315–322. https://doi.org/10.1016/j.jadohealth.2019.03.021
17. Phillips II G, Wang X, Ruprecht MM, et al. Associations between HIV testing and consent policies among sexually active adolescents: differences by sexual behavior. *AIDS Care.* 2022;34(7): 862–868. https://doi.org/10.1080/09540121. 2021.1991878
18. Cordoba E, Kuhns LM, Radix A, Hirsh S. Are state-level HIV testing policies for minors associated with HIV testing behavior and awareness of home-based HIV testing in young men who have sex with men? *J Adolesc Health.* 2022;70(6): 902–909. https://doi.org/10.1016/j.jadohealth. 2021.12.023
19. Culp L, Caucci L. State adolescent consent laws and implications for HIV pre-exposure prophylaxis. *Am J Prev Med.* 2013;44(1 suppl 2):S119–S124. https://doi.org/10.1016/j.amepre.2012.09.044
20. Centers for Disease Control and Prevention. State laws that enable a minor to provide informed consent to receive HIV and STD services. 2021. Available at: https://www.cdc.gov/hiv/policies/law/states/minors.html. Accessed March 15, 2022.
21. Boonstra H, Nash E. Minors and the right to consent to health care. *Guttmacher Report on Public Policy.* Available at: https://www.guttmacher.org/sites/default/files/article_files/gr030404.pdf. Accessed March 15, 2022.
22. Ford CA, Skiles MP, English A, et al. Minor consent and delivery of adolescent vaccines. *J Adolesc Health.* 2014;54(2):183–189. https://doi.org/10.1016/j.jadohealth.2013.07.028
23. English A, Shaw FE, McCauley MM, Fishbein DB. Legal basis of consent for health care and vaccination for adolescents. *Pediatrics.* 2008;121(suppl 1): S85–S87. https://doi.org/10.1542/peds.2007-1115J
24. English A, Bass L, Boyle AD, Eshragh F. *State Minor Consent Laws: A Summary.* 3rd ed. San Francisco, CA: Center for Adolescent Health & the Law; 2010.
25. English A, Gold RB, Nash E, Levine J. Confidentiality for individuals insured as dependents: a review of state laws and policies. Guttmacher Institute. 2012. Available at: https://www.guttmacher.org/report/confidentiality-individuals-insured-dependents-review-state-laws-and-policies. Accessed March 23, 2022.
26. Guttmacher Institute. Minors' access to STI services as of March 1, 2022. 2022. Available at: https://www.guttmacher.org/state-policy/explore/minors-access-sti-services. Accessed March 23, 2022.
27. National Alliance of State and Territorial AIDS Directors. Minor consent and confidentiality laws for HIV treatment and PrEP. 2022. Available at: https://nastad.org/sites/default/files/2022-02/PDF_Minor_Consent_and_Confidentiality_Laws.pdf. Accessed March 24, 2022.
28. Anderson ED, Tremper C, Thomas S, Wagenaar AC. Measuring statutory law and regulations for empirical research. In: Wagenaar AC, Burris SC, eds. *Public Health Law Research: Theory and Methods.* San Francisco, CA: Wiley; 2013:237–260.
29. Gaines DE. Md. lawmakers pass bill giving youth access to HIV-prevention drug without parental consent. *WTOPnews.* March 27, 2019. Available at: https://wtop.com/maryland/2019/03/md-lawmakers-pass-bill-giving-youth-access-to-hiv-prevention-drug-without-parental-consent. Accessed March 24, 2022.
30. Nelson KM, Skinner A, Underhill K. Minor consent laws for sexually transmitted infection and HIV services. *JAMA.* 2022;328(7):674–676. https://doi.org/10.1001/jama.2022.10777
31. Alexander TS. Human immunodeficiency virus diagnostic testing: 30 years of evolution. *Clin Vaccine Immunol.* 2016;23(4):249–253. https://doi.org/10.1128/CVI.00053-16
32. Brandt AM. *No Magic Bullet: A Social History of Venereal Disease in the United States Since 1880.* Exp ed. New York, NY: Oxford University Press; 1987.
33. Allyn D. *Make Love, Not War: The Sexual Revolution: An Unfettered History.* 1st ed. New York, NY: Routledge; 2001.
34. Huntington C, Scott E. Conceptualizing legal childhood in the twenty-first century. *Mich Law Rev.* 2020;118(7):1371–1458. https://doi.org/10.36644/mlr.118.7.conceptualization
35. Alker J, Pham O. Nation's progress on children's health coverage reverses course. Georgetown University Health Policy Institute: Centers for Children and Families. 2018. Available at: https://ccf.georgetown.edu/wp-content/uploads/2018/11/UninsuredKids2018_Final_asof1128743pm.pdf. Accessed April 5, 2019.

Overview of the 2019 National Health Interview Survey Questionnaire Redesign

Benjamin Zablotsky, PhD, Sarah E. Lessem, PhD, Renee M. Gindi, PhD, Aaron K. Maitland, PhD, James M. Dahlhamer, PhD, and Stephen J. Blumberg, PhD

Data System. Federal health surveys, like the National Health Interview Survey (NHIS), represent important surveillance mechanisms for collecting timely, representative data that can be used to monitor the health and health care of the US population.

Data Collection/Processing. Conducted by the National Center for Health Statistics (NCHS), NHIS uses an address-based, complex clustered sample of housing units, yielding data representative of the civilian noninstitutionalized US population. Survey redesigns that reduce survey length and eliminate proxy reporting may reduce respondent burden and increase participation. Such were goals in 2019, when NCHS implemented a redesigned NHIS questionnaire that also focused on topics most relevant and appropriate for surveillance of child and adult health.

Data Analysis/Dissemination. Public-use microdata files and selected health estimates and detailed documentation are released online annually.

Public Health Implications. Declining response rates may lead to biased estimates and weaken users' ability to make valid conclusions from the data, hindering public health efforts. The 2019 NHIS questionnaire redesign was associated with improvements in the survey's response rate, declines in respondent burden, and increases in data quality and survey relevancy. (*Am J Public Health*. 2023;113(4): 408–415. https://doi.org/10.2105/AJPH.2022.307197)

AJPH April 2023, Vol 113, No. 4

The health landscape is in constant flux, with changes in the types and availability of insurance, new places to access care, and novel public health concerns. Data from health surveys are frequently used by policymakers and researchers to set public health agendas and allocate resources.[1] Therefore, survey content needs to reflect the ever-changing health landscape, including changing priorities of sponsoring groups or agencies. In addition, declining survey response rates challenge key assumptions about the representativeness of recruited survey samples.[2] Low response rates may lead to biased estimates and weaken users' ability to make valid conclusions from the data,[2] hindering data used for informing public health efforts.

The National Health Interview Survey (NHIS) has provided data on the nation's health for more than 65 years. The last major redesign of the NHIS questionnaire occurred in 1997 when the survey moved from paper-and-pencil administration to computer-assisted personal interviewing. It "was undertaken because interviews were too long; new or different kinds of information were needed, including better measures of health status and chronic conditions."[3(p509)] The 1997–2018 NHIS questionnaire, sample design, and data collection procedures are available online at https://www.cdc.gov/nchs/nhis/1997-2018.htm.

During the 2 decades following the 1997 redesign, similar concerns about relevance and interview procedures emerged. Decreasing relevance and increasing burden are associated with lower response rates.[4,5] Lower response rates may be linked to response bias and lower data quality.[6] Therefore, the NHIS underwent another major questionnaire redesign for the 2019 survey period, with the goals of reducing respondent burden and increasing survey relevancy and ultimately increasing response rates and data quality.

In this article, we provide key elements of this redesign, particularly a commitment to reducing survey length and eliminating proxy reporting, which, in turn, reduces measurement error and improves data quality.[7,8] In addition, we evaluate whether the redesign achieved its goals by examining quantitative metrics (e.g., response rates, survey length) and established data quality dimensions, including relevancy, accuracy, and reliability.[9] To assist longtime NHIS users, we note major differences from the 1997–2018 NHIS design. We conclude by discussing the public health implications of improved federal health survey data and the continued need for evaluation of the NHIS redesign.

DATA SYSTEM

NHIS is a household survey conducted by the National Center for Health Statistics (NCHS). NCHS is part of the Centers for Disease Control and Prevention (CDC) within the Department of Health and Human Services (DHHS). The NHIS has been fielded continuously since 1957 with periodic updates of survey content and methods.

Purpose

The NHIS is a principal source of health information about the US civilian noninstitutionalized population. NHIS collects data about health insurance, functioning and disability, social determinants of health, and other topics.

Public Health Significance

The NHIS supports DHHS priorities by establishing national benchmarks, monitoring progress toward agency milestone objectives (e.g., Healthy People),[10] and providing nationally representative data on a variety of topics. It is widely used in epidemiological and policy analyses to identify the number and demographics of people with various health conditions, understand the barriers individuals face in accessing and using health care, and evaluate federal health programs.[10]

The NHIS must undergo periodic redesigns to ensure that its content remains relevant while addressing emerging public health topic areas. Questionnaire redesigns allow for alignment with changing DHHS and other public health priorities and may lead to surveys that are more relevant to respondents. This, in turn, may increase participation because of interest in survey topic areas and reduced perceived burden of the survey.

DATA COLLECTION/ PROCESSING

The US Census Bureau is the contracted data collection agent for the NHIS, with 650 to 750 interviewers nationally collecting data. The NHIS is conducted by using computer-assisted personal interviewing, either through face-to-face interviewing in the respondents' homes or over the telephone. In-person interviewing is preferred, but a telephone interview may be conducted when the respondent requests one or when in-person interviewing is infeasible before the required completion date.

Population and Geographic Coverage

The target population for the NHIS is the civilian noninstitutionalized population residing within the 50 states and the District of Columbia. The NHIS sample excludes active-duty military personnel; people living on military bases, in long-term-care institutions, or in correctional facilities; unhoused individuals; and US nationals living abroad. Residents of households and noninstitutional group quarters (e.g., group homes) are eligible for the survey.

Rostering and Interviewing Participants

As the NHIS sampling frame consists of addresses rather than individuals, the interviewer first asks 1 household respondent to name and provide demographic information about all people living at the address. After the roster, 1 adult ("sample adult," herein referred to as "SA") and, in households with children, 1 child ("sample child," herein referred to as "SC") are randomly selected for detailed health-related questions.

From 1997 to 2018, the NHIS included a family questionnaire after the household roster and before the SA or SC interview. The family questionnaire asked about the family and the health of each family member. In the redesigned NHIS, the family questionnaire was eliminated to reduce interview length and proxy reporting. Family-level content is now collected within the SA or SC interview, and no health questions are asked about other family members. The instrument is optimized to only ask family-level questions of the first respondent when the SA and SC are in the same family. When the SA and SC are in different families, family-level questions are asked in both interviews. For more information about changes to the questionnaire structure, reference the 2019 Survey Description documentation.[11]

Unit of Data Collection and Sample Size

The SA and SC are the main units of data collection in the redesigned NHIS. Approximately 30 000 SA and 9000 SC interviews are completed annually. Sample size may vary annually depending on budget and supplementary funding.

Surveillance Design and Frequency of Data Collection

Because the NHIS uses in-person interviewing, the costs of interviewing a nationally representative simple random sample of households and noninstitutional group quarters would be prohibitive. To keep survey operations manageable, affordable, and timely, the NHIS uses geographically clustered sampling techniques to select the sample of dwelling units for the NHIS. Data collection on the NHIS is continuous (January–December), and each month's sample is nationally representative.

Sample areas are reselected every 10 years to account for changes in the distribution of the US population.[12] The 2016–2025 NHIS sampling plan was designed with results of the 2010 Decennial Census.[13] NHIS uses an address-based sample—interviewers travel to selected properties rather than tracking down persons. Commercial address lists are supplemented by address lists developed by Census canvassing operations.

Ethical Procedures

NHIS is a public health surveillance activity excluded from the regulatory requirements of 45 CFR 46; procedures and protocols are reviewed and approved by the NCHS Ethics Review Board to protect the rights and welfare of participants. Before the interview, each sample household is mailed an "advance letter" describing the NHIS. Interviewers arrive at the household, offer another copy of the advance letter to respondents, and obtain their verbal consent to participate. Parents or guardians provide consent and answer questions on behalf of their children.

National Health Interview Survey Funding

While the majority of NHIS data collection costs are covered by NCHS's appropriated funding, the NHIS serves as a platform to meet the needs of other federal agencies who provide additional funds for survey content. Sponsored content helps ensure that the redesigned NHIS questionnaire stays relevant in a continually changing health landscape. The amount of content added each year is limited to reduce burden. Sponsored content may be annual or periodic.

Key Data Elements and Data Quality and Editing

During the 2019 redesign efforts, questions from the most recent NHIS questionnaires were reviewed to address survey length and respondent burden. Categories of questions dropped from the redesigned NHIS questionnaire were those (1) about rare conditions and services (< 2% prevalence), (2) for which data were better collected elsewhere (e.g., federal surveys or administrative records), (3) that did not align with DHHS priorities, and (4) that were rarely used (based on public comment solicitations and literature reviews of published findings).

In the redesigned NHIS, some questions are included annually while others are included with fixed periodicity (e.g., every other year, 2 out of 3 years). Introducing a larger number of topics enhances survey relevancy. Including them periodically reduces annual survey length and respondent burden. Similar topics are addressed for both SA and SC interviews each year.

Topic prioritization and survey relevancy. Topic areas that are well-measured through household interviews, produce reliable estimates for demographic subgroups using 1 or 2 years of data, and are used for long-term monitoring, such as leading causes of morbidity and mortality and associated risk factors (e.g., social determinants), were prioritized in the redesigned NHIS. Topics featured in the DHHS Strategic Plan 2018–2022[14] and Healthy People 2020 leading health indicators[11] were also prioritized.

NCHS engaged stakeholders on the redesign by meeting with staff across CDC centers, agency partners, federal interagency working groups, and professional associations, and sought input about the redesign through online outreach and through *Federal Register* notices. NCHS also invited technical experts in child health, income, pain, injury, and opioid use to provide feedback on topic relevancy and efficient measurement approaches.

Another way the redesigned NHIS stays relevant is by reserving limited space for NCHS to add emerging content on key DHHS priorities. Content is considered emerging if it is experimental (having never, or not recently, been fielded on the NHIS) or is of growing interest (but long-term monitoring may be unnecessary). A focused effort on including questions in a survey that reflects the current health landscape naturally allows for an alignment with changing departmental priorities, and it may lead to a survey that is more relevant for respondents. Previous research has found respondents who have a strong interest in questionnaire content are more attentive,[15] which can lead to less burden and better-quality data.[16,17] For more information on NHIS redesign priorities and public outreach activities, visit https://www.cdc.gov/nchs/nhis/2019_quest_redesign.htm.

Question validity and reliability. When developing questions on new topics, survey methodologists looked for validated health scales and questions from other surveys that had undergone testing and been found effective at capturing the construct of interest. For example, the redesign incorporated the validated Washington Group Extended Set on Functioning[18] and the Washington Group/UNICEF Module on Child Functioning[19] to assess disability. This process increased the relevance of the NHIS and provided data coherence, allowing for standardized comparisons across different countries and languages.[20] When no appropriate question could be found, questions were developed internally. All new questions were tested at the Collaborating Center for Questionnaire Design and Evaluation Research within NCHS, which used cognitive interviewing to evaluate survey questions, uncover the constructs questions measure, and identify potentially confusing questions.[21]

As part of the redesign, efforts were also made to decrease the question difficulty by shortening question length, lowering reading level, and eliminating medical terminology when possible. Combined, these reductions in question difficulty and cognitive burden were aimed to improve data quality.[22]

Approximately 5% of NHIS interviews are conducted in Spanish. Before the redesign, there was no standardized approach for translating questions into Spanish, with questions translated by different people. This resulted in inconsistent wordings, styles, and overall quality. In the redesign, all English questions were translated or retranslated with more consistent wording and syntax.

Weighting. As part of the redesign, weighting processes were updated to better address potential nonresponse bias,[23] further enhancing data quality by improving the accuracy and reliability of NHIS estimates. Multilevel logistic regression models with variables from multiple sources were used to predict response propensities, and raking procedures included more variables for calibration to population control totals.

Edits to protect confidentiality. The NCHS has strict procedures to prevent disclosure of survey respondents' identities. In addition to restricting geographical information, data appearing on publicly released files are edited to minimize the potential for inadvertent disclosure of confidential information. Data from some questions have been coarsened, including top and bottom coding and collapsing response categories. Data from multiple questions may be collapsed into 1 variable, and statistical noise may be added at either or both the variable level and record level to protect confidentiality.

Data imputation. To address high nonresponse rates to questions on total family income, files containing imputations of family income and income-to-poverty ratio (as continuous and categorical top-coded variables) are made available annually. As part of the redesign effort, to improve data quality, NCHS now includes 10 imputed data files (compared with 5 used previously) to reflect recent literature[24] that recommends increasing the number of imputations to 10 or higher to establish scientific integrity and produce more efficient estimates for a wide variety of analyses. Additional information on the imputation method for total family income and how to use imputed values is available at http://www.cdc.gov/nchs/nhis.htm.

DATA ANALYSIS/ DISSEMINATION

The annual NHIS data release now includes a data file and an imputed income file for both the SA and SC, as well as a paradata file. Unlike previous data releases, there is no longer a person or family data file.

Data Release Accessibility

Data users interested in learning more about the purpose, goals, and history of the NHIS, or in downloading public data sets, codebooks, and survey documentation, should visit the NHIS Web site (https://www.cdc.gov/nchs/nhis.htm). Data users should read the Survey Description documents, which include sample sizes and provide instructions to properly account for the NHIS complex survey design. NHIS public-use data files since 1963 are available online. Analysts interested in working with restricted data may apply for access through the NCHS Research Data Center. For more information, see https://www.cdc.gov/rdc.

Throughout each year, NCHS releases a series of reports in various forms (e.g., NCHS Data Briefs,[25] National Health Statistics Reports[26]). NCHS also provides an interactive data query system that produces tables and charts for key indicators, nationally or by select demographics (known as Summary Health Statistics[27]). In addition, NHIS has an Early Release program that provides key health estimates and preliminary microdata files on an expedited schedule.

Interpretation Issues

Research shows that self-respondents and proxy respondents give different answers to health questions.[28] While proxy respondents may report accurately on observable events, such as physical tasks of daily living, they cannot always accurately answer questions about chronic physical and mental health conditions and pain.[9,28] The elimination of the family interview virtually eliminated proxy reporting for adults (previously 55% of all responses for adults in the family were through a proxy). Proxy health-related information about adults is only collected if the SA is unable to answer for themselves (< 2% of all interviews).

Adding, dropping, or rotating questions may affect question order and context. These changes may affect responses by changing respondents' interpretations of the questions. However, to minimize this impact, new questions were embedded into existing sections when appropriate. When this was not possible, new questions with similar content were grouped together.

Given these redesign changes detailed previously, many data users may ask if it is appropriate to trend data before and after the NHIS redesign, particularly as it relates to content previously in the family interview. NCHS evaluated a set of 19 Early Release indicators measured in the 2018 and 2019 NHIS to examine the impact of the weighting and questionnaire redesign on the comparability of estimates.[29] The report showed variable results, although for 6 out of the 19 indicators neither the questionnaire nor the updated weighted approach appeared to have an impact. NCHS will continue to evaluate the ability to conduct trend analyses across the redesign period and monitor the ability to trend between survey years moving forward. Users should be aware of this issue when analyzing years that span the redesign.

Linkage Capabilities

NHIS is part of the Data Linkage Program at NCHS, which links NCHS survey data with data from vital and other administrative records, including the National Death Index, the Centers for Medicare and Medicaid Services, the Department of Housing and Urban Development, and the Department of Veterans Affairs. These linked data are available for NHIS participants who have provided consent, as well as the necessary personally identifiable information, and for whom NCHS was able to match with the administrative records source. Linked data allow richer analyses of the survey data by augmenting the information collected from the surveys with vital or administrative data that let researchers examine factors that influence disability, chronic disease, health care utilization, morbidity, and mortality.[30]

Key Sources

- NHIS Web site: https://www.cdc.gov/nchs/nhis.htm
- 2019 NHIS Survey Description: https://ftp.cdc.gov/pub/Health_Statistics/NCHS/Dataset_Documentation/NHIS/2019/srvydesc-508.pdf
- 2019 NHIS Weighting Report: https://ftp.cdc.gov/pub/Health_Statistics/NCHS/Dataset_Documentation/NHIS/2019/nonresponse-report-508.pdf

IMPLICATIONS

The response rates for the SA and SC interviews were calculated by first dividing the number of completed and sufficient partial SA or SC interviews, respectively, by the number of eligible SAs or SCs, respectively, and then multiplying by the household roster competition rate, which is the percentage of interviewed and nonresponding (including noncontacts and refusals) households with a completed roster.[11,31] These served as key metrics in evaluating the redesign impact, along with factors that may have longer-term impacts on response rate including survey length, item nonresponse, and respondent burden.

Given the impact of the COVID-19 pandemic on survey operations,[32] response rates and other metrics are not presented for the 2020 NHIS.

Response Rate

After the first year of data collection, differences between the redesigned and previous NHIS were evaluated by examining response rate and survey length (pooling 2016–2018 given survey-length fluctuations). There was a significant increase in the SA interview response rate in the 2019 NHIS (59.1% vs 53.1%), while SC interview response rate (59.1% vs 59.2%; Figure 1) and overall response rate (61.1% vs 64.2%) were comparable.

Survey Length

Longer questionnaires are associated with higher respondent fatigue, which

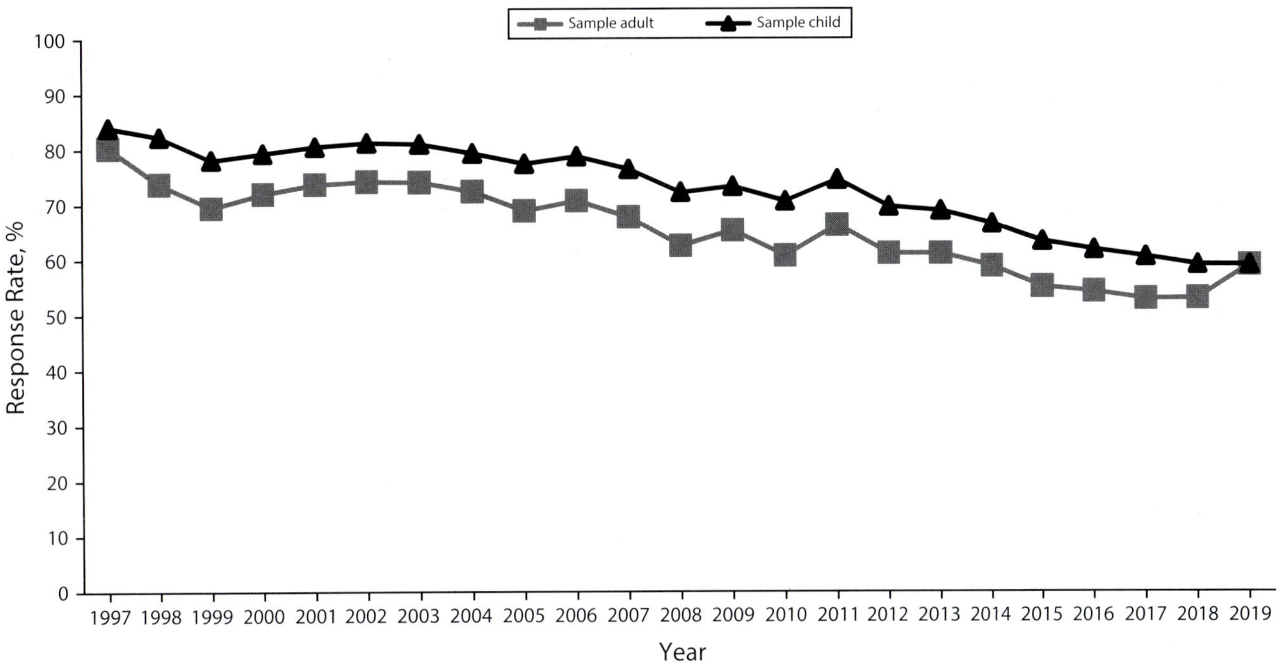

FIGURE 1— Sample Adult and Sample Child Response Rates: United States, National Health Interview Survey, 1997–2019

Note. Final sample adult (SA) and sample child (SC) response rates were calculated by dividing the number of completed and sufficient partial SA or SC interviews, respectively, by the number of eligible SA and SC, respectively, and then multiplying this quotient by the percentage of eligible households with completed rosters (household roster completion rate).

AJPH April 2023, Vol 113, No. 4

can lead to greater missing data as respondents become less attentive, answer questions faster, and show smaller variability in their responses.[33]

The 2019 survey had a median length of 48.0 minutes per completed interview (n = 30 532), significantly shorter than before (72.5 minutes; n = 81 031). Most of this reduction can be attributed to the elimination of the family interview (median time of 18.4 minutes in 2016–2018). The rostering component of the 2019 and 2016–2018 NHIS were comparable in length (3.0 vs 4.1 minutes), while the 2019 SA interview was shorter than the 2016–2018 SA interview (33.7 vs 37.9 minutes), and the 2019 SC interview was longer than the 2016–2018 SC interview (15.8 vs 11.3 minutes). The longer SC interview can be attributed to the addition of topic areas to create a more comprehensive picture of a child's health and environment.

Item Nonresponse

Data quality is a multidimensional construct,[10] lending itself to an array of metrics for evaluation. Many of the NHIS redesign efforts were focused on enhancing data accuracy and reliability of survey responses. Reducing survey length and proxy reporting has been shown to reduce item nonresponse.[34] Changes to both weighting and multiple imputation procedures during the redesign were meant to address

TABLE 1— Percent Distribution of Item Nonresponse in Sample Adult and Sample Child Interviews: United States, National Health Interview Survey, 2018–2019

	Sample Adult, %		Sample Child, %	
Percent Missingness	2018 (n = 25 417)	2019 (n = 31 997)	2018 (n = 8 629)	2019 (n = 9 193)
0	27.1	33.4[a]	79.0	86.7[b]
> 0 to < 1.5	47.7	46.5[a]	6.1	7.4[b]
≥ 1.5	25.2	20.1[a]	14.9	5.9[b]

[a]Significantly different from 2018 sample adult by logistic regression ($P < .05$).
[b]Significantly different from 2018 sample child by logistic regression ($P < .05$).

TABLE 2— Percent Distribution of Respondent Perception of Burden by Questionnaire: United States, National Health Interview Survey, October–December 2018

	Previous Questionnaire (n = 3926), %	Redesigned Questionnaire (n = 3924), %
Not at all	52.9	62.5[a]
A little	29.6	25.6[a]
Moderately	12.2	8.5[a]
Very	3.2	2.2[a]
Extremely	2.1	1.2[a]

Note. In total, 11.9% of respondents in the redesigned questionnaire found the questionnaire moderately to extremely burdensome, significantly less than the 17.5% of respondents in the previous questionnaire ($P < .05$).

[a]Significantly different from the previous questionnaire by logistic regression ($P < .05$).

nonresponse, be it at the survey or item level. Doing such reduces the potential for systematic bias in responses and may produce larger sample sizes for given items.

Considering just items included in both the 2019 and 2018 SA interviews, the percentage of interviews with any item nonresponse was significantly lower in the redesigned NHIS (66.4% vs 72.9%). Similarly, the percentage of SC interviews with any item nonresponse was significantly lower in the redesigned NHIS (13.3% vs 21.0%; Table 1).

Respondent Burden

The burden experienced by respondents completing the NHIS can be tied to several factors, including item difficulty, sensitivity, and questionnaire length.[35] From October to December 2018, NCHS conducted a test to determine whether health estimates and respondents' perception of burden differed between the 2018 NHIS and the redesigned NHIS. A split-sample comparison was conducted in which sample addresses were randomly assigned to receive either the 2018 NHIS or the redesigned NHIS. This overlap in data collection served as a "bridge" between the 2 designs. Differences in health estimates were identified for several key indicators (e.g., unmet needs for medical and mental health care because of cost) and have been reported elsewhere.[29]

After completing the survey, respondents were asked, "How burdensome was this survey to you?" A total of 11.9% of respondents assigned to the redesigned questionnaire reported that they found the interview to be moderately to extremely burdensome, significantly less than the 17.5% of respondents who were assigned to the 2018 questionnaire (Table 2).

Conclusions

Federal health surveys such as NHIS are an important surveillance mechanism for collecting timely and representative data that are used to monitor the health and health care of the US population. Federal surveys must remain flexible to accommodating new questions on emerging issues that help to fulfill departmental and agency data needs and current missions and priorities. In some instances, like that of the NHIS, this may require redesigning the survey to ensure it remains relevant and of high quality and produces low burden for respondents, while incorporating advances in survey methodology to reduce nonresponse. By doing such, policymakers and researchers can continue to rely on federal statistics for making timely and informed public health decisions. Efforts to evaluate these elements must be ongoing, drawing from multiple years of data as they become available, and responding and adapting to changes in the survey climate. AJPH

ABOUT THE AUTHORS

Benjamin Zablotsky, Renee M. Gindi, Aaron K. Maitland, James M. Dahlhamer, and Stephen J. Blumberg are with the National Center for Health Statistics, Centers for Disease Control and Prevention, Hyattsville, MD. Sarah E. Lessem is with RTI International, Washington, DC.

Note. The findings and conclusions in this report are those of the authors and do not necessarily represent the official position of the Centers for Disease Control and Prevention or RTI International.

CORRESPONDENCE

Correspondence should be sent to Benjamin Zablotsky, PhD, National Center for Health Statistics, 3311 Toledo Rd, Hyattsville, MD 20782 (e-mail: bzablotsky@cdc.gov). Reprints can be ordered at https://ajph.org by clicking the "Reprints" link.

PUBLICATION INFORMATION

Full Citation: Zablotsky B, Lessem SE, Gindi RM, Maitland AK, Dahlhamer JM, Blumberg SJ. Overview of the 2019 National Health Interview Survey questionnaire redesign. *Am J Public Health*. 2023; 113(4):408–415.

Acceptance Date: December 2, 2022.

DOI: https://doi.org/10.2105/AJPH.2022.307197

CONTRIBUTORS

B. Zablotsky, S. E. Lessem, and R. M. Gindi conceptualized the study and drafted the article. A. K. Maitland, J. M. Dahlhamer, and S. J. Blumberg provided significant input, review, and editing. All authors read and approved the final version of the article.

CONFLICTS OF INTEREST

The authors have no conflicts of interest relevant to this article to disclose.

HUMAN PARTICIPANT PROTECTION

Centers for Disease Control and Prevention research on human participants complies with Department of Health and Human Services Policy for Protection of Human Research Subjects. All National Health Interview Survey procedures and protocols have been reviewed and approved by the National Center for Health Statistics Research Ethics Review Board.

REFERENCES

1. Blewett LA, Call KT, Turner J, Hest R. Data resources for conducting health services and policy research. *Annu Rev Public Health.* 2018;39(1):437–452. https://doi.org/10.1146/annurev-publhealth-040617-013544
2. National Research Council. *Panel on a Research Agenda for the Future of Social Science Data Collection, Committee on National Statistics.* Washington, DC: The National Academies Press; 2013.
3. Fowler FJ Jr. The redesign of the National Health Interview Survey. *Public Health Rep.* 1996;111(6):508–511.
4. Groves RM, Presser S, Dipko S. The role of topic interest in survey participation decisions. *Public Opin Q.* 2004;68(1):2–31. https://doi.org/10.1093/poq/nfh002
5. Andreadis I, Kartsounidou E. The impact of splitting a long online questionnaire on data quality. *Survey Res Methods.* 2020;14(1):31–42. https://doi.org/10.18148/SRM/2020.V14I1.7294
6. Deutskens E, De Ruyter K, Wetzels M, Oosterveld P. Response rate and response quality of internet-based surveys: an experimental study. *Mark Lett.* 2004;15(1):21–36. https://doi.org/10.1023/B:MARK.0000021968.86465.00
7. Peytchev A, Peytcheva E. Reduction of measurement error due to survey length: evaluation of the split questionnaire design approach. *Survey Res Methods.* 2017;11(4):361–368. https://doi.org/10.18148/SRM/2017.V11I4.7145
8. Andresen EM, Vahle VJ, Lollar D. Proxy reliability: health-related quality of life (HRQoL) measures for people with disability. *Qual Life Res.* 2001;10(7):609–619. https://doi.org/10.1023/A:1013187903591
9. Federal Committee on Statistical Methodology. A framework for data quality. FCSM 20-04. September 2020. Available at: https://nces.ed.gov/fcsm/pdf/FCSM.20.04_A_Framework_for_Data_Quality.pdf. Accessed January 12, 2023.
10. US Department of Health and Human Services, Office of Disease Prevention and Health Promotion. Healthy People 2020. Available at: https://www.cdc.gov/nchs/healthy_people/hp2020.htm. Accessed October 12, 2020.
11. National Center for Health Statistics. Survey Description, National Health Interview Survey, 2019. 2020. Available at: https://ftp.cdc.gov/pub/Health_Statistics/NCHS/Dataset_Documentation/NHIS/2019/srvydesc-508.pdf. Accessed October 12, 2022.
12. Parsons VL, Moriarity C, Jonas K, et al. Design and estimation for the National Health Interview Survey, 2006–2015. National Center for Health Statistics. *Vital Health Stat 2.* 2014;(165):1–53.
13. Moriarity C, Parsons VL, Jonas K, Schar BG, Bose J, Bramlett MD. Sample design and estimation structures for the National Health Interview Survey, 2016–2025. National Center for Health Statistics. *Vital Health Stat 1.* 2022;(191):1–30.
14. Department of Health and Human Services. Overview: HHS Strategic Plan, FY 2018–2022. Available at: https://www.hhs.gov/about/strategic-plan/overview/index.html#overview. Accessed September 29, 2022.
15. Couper MP. Survey introductions and data quality. *Public Opin Q.* 1997;61(2):317–338. https://doi.org/10.1086/297797
16. Silber H, Danner D, Rammstedt B. The impact of respondent attentiveness on reliability and validity. *Int J Soc Res Methodol.* 2019;22(2):153–164. https://doi.org/10.1080/13645579.2018.1507378
17. Crawford SD, Couper MP, Lamias MJ. Web surveys: perceptions of burden. *Soc Sci Comput Rev.* 2001;19(2):146–162. https://doi.org/10.1177/089443930101900202
18. Washington Group on Disability Statistics. Washington Group Extended Set on Functioning. Available at: https://www.washingtongroup-disability.com/question-sets/wg-extended-set-on-functioning-wg-es. Accessed May 31, 2020.
19. Washington Group on Disability Statistics. Washington Group/UNICEF Module on Child Functioning. Available at: https://www.washingtongroup-disability.com/question-sets/wg-unicef-child-functioning-module-cfm. Accessed May 31, 2020.
20. Madans JH, Loeb M. Methods to improve international comparability of census and survey measures of disability. *Disabil Rehabil.* 2013;35(13):1070–1073. https://doi.org/10.3109/09638288.2012.720353
21. Miller K, Willson S, Chepp V, Padilla JL. *Cognitive Interviewing Methodology.* Hoboken, NJ: Wiley; 2014. https://doi.org/10.1002/9781118838860
22. Robinson SB, Leonard KF. *Designing Quality Survey Questions.* Los Angeles, CA: Sage Publications; 2018.
23. Bramlett MD, Dahlhamer JM, Bose J, Blumberg SJ. New procedures for nonresponse adjustments to the 2019 National Health Interview Survey sampling weights. September 2020. Available at: https://ftp.cdc.gov/pub/Health_Statistics/NCHS/Dataset_Documentation/NHIS/2019/nonresponse-report-508.pdf. Accessed September 29, 2022.
24. Van Buuren S. *Flexible Imputation of Missing Data.* 2nd ed. New York, NY: Chapman and Hall/CRC; 2018. https://doi.org/10.1201/9780429492259
25. National Center for Health Statistics. Data Briefs from the National Health Interview Survey. Available at: https://www.cdc.gov/nchs/nhis/nhis_db.htm. Accessed May 31, 2022.
26. National Center for Health Statistics. Reports from the National Health Interview Survey. Available at: https://www.cdc.gov/nchs/nhis/nhis_nhsr.htm. Accessed May 31, 2022.
27. National Center for Health Statistics. Interactive Data Query Systems. Available at: https://www.cdc.gov/nchs/nhis/shs.htm. Accessed May 31, 2022.
28. Lee S, Mathiowetz N, Tourangeau R. Perceptions of disability: the effect of self and proxy response. *J Off Stat.* 2004;20:671–686.
29. National Center for Health Statistics. Preliminary evaluation of the impact of the 2019 National Health Interview Survey questionnaire redesign and weighting adjustments on Early Release Program estimates. September 2020. Available at: https://www.cdc.gov/nchs/data/nhis/earlyrelease/EReval202009-508.pdf. Accessed May 31, 2022.
30. Golden C, Mirel LB. Enhancement of health surveys with data linkage. In: Chun AY, Larsen MD, Durrant G, Reiter JP, eds. *Administrative Records for Survey Methodology.* Hoboken, NJ: John Wiley and Sons Inc; 2021:271–292. https://doi.org/10.1002/9781119272076.ch11
31. American Association for Public Opinion Research. *Standard Definitions: Final Disposition of Case Codes and Outcomes Rates for Surveys.* 9th ed. 2016. Available at: https://www-archive.aapor.org/AAPOR_Main/media/publications/Standard-Definitions20169theditionfinal.pdf. Accessed January 12, 2023.
32. Blumberg SJ, Parker JD, Moyer BC. National Health Interview Survey, COVID-19, and online data collection platforms: adaptations, tradeoffs, and new directions. *Am J Public Health.* 2021;111(12):2167–2175. https://doi.org/10.2105/AJPH.2021.306516
33. Galesic M, Bosnjak M. Effects of questionnaire length on participation and indicators of response quality in a web survey. *Public Opin Q.* 2009;73(2):349–360. https://doi.org/10.1093/poq/nfp031
34. De Leeuw ED, van der Zouwen J. Data quality in telephone and face-to-face surveys: a comparative meta-analysis. In: Groves RM, Biemer PP, Lyberg LE, et al, eds. *Telephone Survey Methodology.* New York, NY: John Wiley and Sons; 1988.
35. Bradburn N. Respondent burden. In: *Proceedings of the Survey Research Methods Section of the American Statistical Association.* Alexandria, VA: American Statistical Association; 1978.

Methamphetamine-Related Mortality in the United States: Co-Involvement of Heroin and Fentanyl, 1999–2021

Rachel A. Hoopsick, PhD, MS, MPH, MCHES, and R. Andrew Yockey, PhD

AJPH April 2023, Vol 113, No. 4

Objectives. To examine trends in methamphetamine-related mortality in the United States from 1999 to 2021 and the extent to which these deaths co-involved heroin or fentanyl.

Methods. We obtained final and provisional data from the CDC WONDER (Centers for Disease Control and Prevention Wide-ranging ONline Data for Epidemiologic Research) multiple causes of death database for deaths that involved methamphetamine and deaths that involved both methamphetamine and heroin or fentanyl mong US residents aged 15 to 74 years. We plotted the age-adjusted methamphetamine-related mortality rate by year and quantified the proportion of deaths with heroin or fentanyl co-involvement. Finally, we used joinpoint regression to quantify trends in the methamphetamine mortality rate and proportion of deaths with heroin or fentanyl co-involvement.

Results. From 1999 to 2021, there was a 50-fold increase in the methamphetamine mortality rate, which was accompanied by an increasing proportion of deaths that co-involved heroin or fentanyl, peaking at 61.2% in 2021.

Conclusions. Unprecedented increases in methamphetamine-related mortality have occurred during the last decade, and an increasing proportion of these deaths co-involved heroin or fentanyl.

Public Health Implications. Stark increases in methamphetamine-related mortality and heroin or fentanyl co-involvement warrant robust harm reduction efforts, especially for people who engage in polysubstance use. (*Am J Public Health*. 2023;113(4):416–419. https://doi.org/10.2105/AJPH.2022.307212)

A staggering increase in drug overdose deaths was observed in the United States in 2020.[1] Moreover, the Centers for Disease Control and Prevention (CDC) reported that 2021 included the deadliest rolling 12-month period for drug overdose deaths on record thus far.[2] Prepandemic data show upward trends in methamphetamine use,[3] methamphetamine and heroin co-use,[4] and methamphetamine-related mortality in the United States.[3] In 2019, more than half of all psychostimulant overdose deaths also involved opioids,[5] suggesting that the second (i.e., heroin) and third (i.e., fentanyl) waves of the opioid overdose crisis may be driving recent methamphetamine-related mortality. Given the steep increases in overall drug overdose mortality observed in 2020 and 2021,[1,2] an updated examination of the trends in methamphetamine-related mortality is warranted. Moreover, it is critical to contextualize these deaths within the ongoing opioid overdose crisis by examining the extent to which methamphetamine-related mortality may be exacerbated by the co-involvement of heroin and fentanyl.

Qualitative data suggest that the co-use of methamphetamine and opioids is motivated by a desire to achieve specific embodied experiences not attained by methamphetamine or opioid use alone.[6] Moreover, a recent qualitative study suggests that there is significant variation in the presentation and severity of stimulant-involved overdoses ("overamping"), which may limit the ability of people who use stimulants to recognize and respond to an overdose.[7] The last 2 decades have also been marked by increased contamination of the unregulated drug supply with fentanyl and fentanyl-related analogs,[8,9] suggesting that intentional and unintentional co-use may be catalyzing methamphetamine-related mortality in the United States. In this descriptive epidemiological analysis, we quantify the trends in methamphetamine-related mortality and the proportion of these deaths that also involved heroin or fentanyl, including time-sensitive changes not captured in prepandemic data.

METHODS

We obtained 1999–2021 death certificate data from the CDC Wide-ranging ONline Data for Epidemiologic Research (WONDER) final (for 1999 through 2020) and provisional (for 2021) multiple causes of death databases.[10] We examined the annual number of deaths involving methamphetamine and the age-adjusted overdose mortality rates per 100 000 population among US residents aged 15 to 74 years. We included causes of death in the following categories (*International Classification of Diseases, 10th Revision* codes): accidental/unintentional poisoning (X40–X44), intentional self-poisoning/suicide (X60–X64), assault/homicide (X85), and undetermined intent (Y10–Y14). In addition, methamphetamine-related deaths included deaths with a contributing cause of poisoning by psychostimulants with abuse potential (T43.6). We then examined what proportion of methamphetamine-related deaths co-involved heroin (T40.1) or other synthetic narcotics (T40.4; i.e., fentanyl and fentanyl-related analogs) each year. As a post hoc analysis for comparison, we also examined the annual number of cocaine-related deaths (T40.5), age-adjusted cocaine mortality rate, and the proportion of cocaine-related deaths that also included heroin or fentanyl over the same time period.

We quantified trends in the age-adjusted methamphetamine mortality rate and proportion of deaths with heroin or fentanyl co-involvement using joinpoint regression, which uses permutation to fit a series of straight lines on a logarithmic scale to aggregated data to estimate annual percent change (APC) trends of variable length and the slopes of these trends (b). We also estimated 95% confidence intervals (CIs) with each APC and reported the corresponding P value. The APC was considered statistically significant if the P value was less than .05. We conducted analyses with Stata/MP version 17.0 (StataCorp LP, College Station, TX) and Joinpoint Regression Program version 4.9.1.0 (National Cancer Institute, Bethesda, MD https://surveillance.cancer.gov/joinpoint/).

RESULTS

From 1999 to 2021, there were 135 433 methamphetamine-related deaths among US residents aged 15 to 74 years, and 42.8% of these deaths also involved heroin or fentanyl. Across these 23 years of data, there was a 58-fold increase in the annual number of methamphetamine-related deaths (545 methamphetamine-related deaths in 1999 vs 32 353 methamphetamine-related deaths in 2021; Figure 1, panel a) and more than a 50-fold increase in the age-adjusted methamphetamine-related mortality rate (0.27 deaths per 100 000 in 1999 vs 13.93 deaths per 100 000 in 2021; Figure 1, panel b). Annual co-involvement of heroin or fentanyl ranged from 7.3% (2005) to 61.2% (2021), with stark increases observed over the last decade. Post hoc analyses suggest there have also been increases in cocaine-related mortality and co-involvement with heroin or fentanyl, but these trends were more variable over time (Figure A, available as a supplement to the online version of this article at http://www.ajph.org).

The age-adjusted methamphetamine-related mortality rate increased annually by 20.1% from 1999 to 2005 (APC = 20.1%; 95% CI = 14.9, 25.6; $P < .001$; $b = 0.18$), remained stable from 2005 to 2008 (APC = −8.6%; 95% CI = −29.7, 18.8; $P > .05$; $b = -0.09$), continued to increase 21.8% annually from 2008 to 2014 (APC = 21.8%; 95% CI = 14.9, 29.1; $P < .001$; $b = 0.20$), and further increased by 32.5% annually from 2014 to 2021 (APC = 32.5%; 95% CI = 28.0, 37.2; $P < .001$; $b = 0.28$). The proportion of methamphetamine-related deaths with heroin or fentanyl co-involvement decreased by 6.6% annually from 1999 to 2005 (APC = −6.6%; 95% CI = −9.4, −3.6; $P < .001$; $b = -0.07$), increased by 8.9% annually from 2005 to 2010 (APC = 8.9%; 95% CI = 2.7, 15.5; $P < .01$; $b = 0.09$), and increased by 17.3% annually from 2010 to 2021 (APC = 17.3%; 95% CI = 15.8, 18.8; $P < .001$; $b = 0.16$).

DISCUSSION

Consistent with overall drug overdose deaths observed in 2020 and 2021,[1,2] our results suggest that methamphetamine-related mortality has accelerated over the last 2 decades, peaking in 2021. Importantly, this was accompanied by a dramatic growth in the percentage of these deaths that co-involved heroin or fentanyl. The proportional increases in methamphetamine-related mortality and illicit opioid involvement suggest that these stimulant deaths are largely driven by polysubstance use. Intentional co-use of stimulants and opioids has increased over time,[4] which appears to be motivated in part by desire, pleasure,

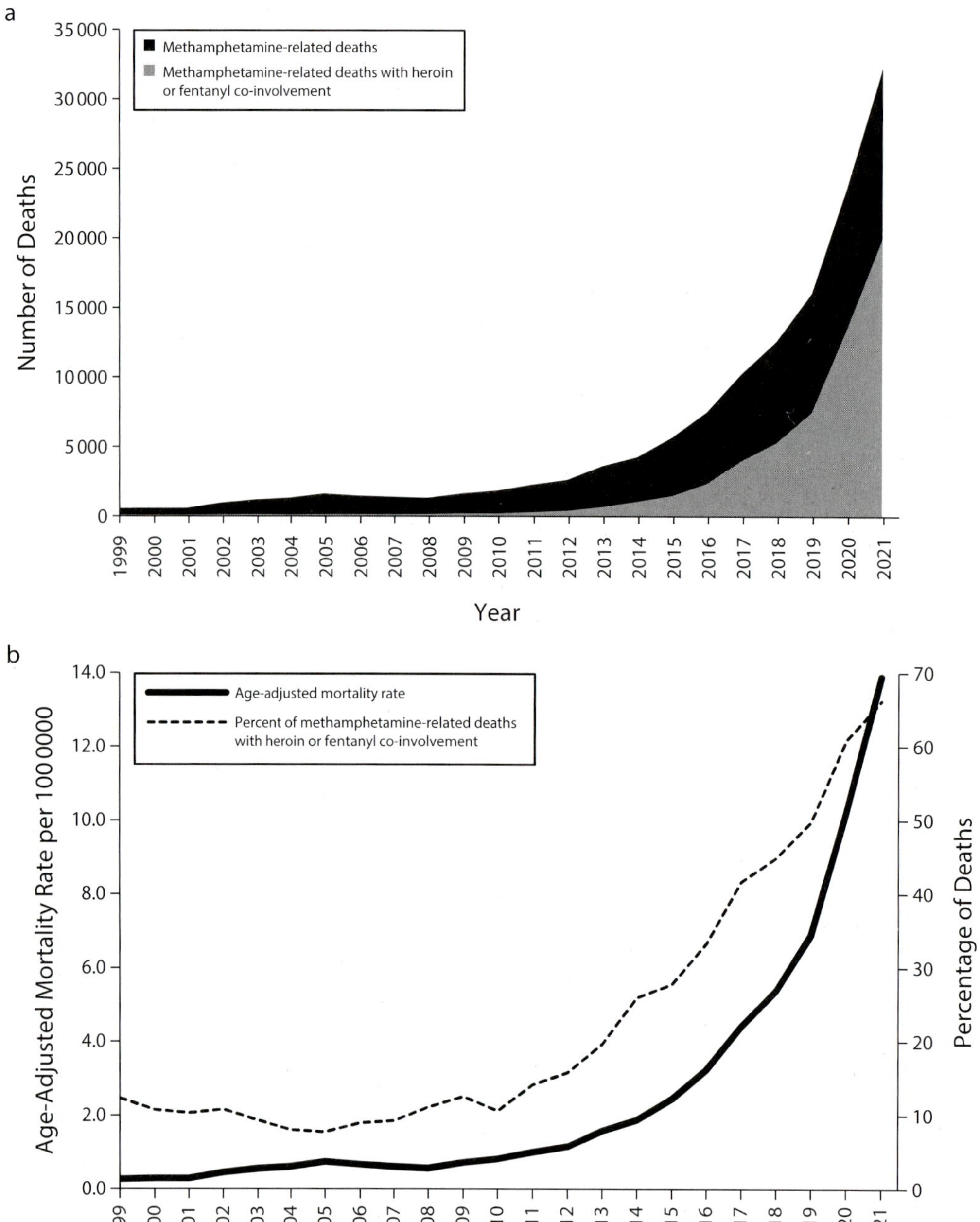

FIGURE 1— Number (a) and Rate (b) of Deaths Involving Methamphetamine and Its Co-Involvement With Heroin or Fentanyl Among People Aged 15–74 Years: CDC WONDER, United States, 1999–2021

Note. CDC WONDER = Centers for Disease Control and Prevention Wide-ranging ONline Data for Epidemiologic Research. Methamphetamine-related deaths included causes of death in the following categories (*International Classification of Diseases, 10th Revision* codes): accidental/unintentional poisoning (X40–X44), intentional self-poisoning/suicide (X60–X64), assault/homicide (X85), and undetermined intent (Y10–Y14) with a contributing cause of poisoning by psychostimulants with abuse potential (T43.6). Methamphetamine-related deaths that involved heroin or fentanyl included deaths with a contributing cause of poisoning by psychostimulants with abuse potential (T43.6) and a contributing cause of poisoning by heroin (T40.1) or other synthetic narcotics (T40.4).

and control.[6] However, the illicit drug supply in the United States has also become increasingly toxic with the adulteration of street opioids and other drugs with fentanyl and fentanyl-related analogs.[8,9]

This study has some limitations. Deaths of nonresidents (e.g., nonresident aliens, nationals living abroad, residents of Puerto Rico, Guam, the Virgin Islands, and other US territories) are not recorded in CDC WONDER[10] and were not included in the current study. Additionally, deaths in which toxicology tests were not performed or were unable to detect the substances examined here were excluded. However, the exclusion of nonresidents and death certificates without drug-specific information is likely to result in an underestimation of methamphetamine-related mortality. Similarly, data for 2021 are provisional and therefore subject to reporting lags, necessitating future updates. Additional research is needed to examine whether there have been any shifts in unique subgroup risks for methamphetamine-related mortality by age, race/ethnicity, and gender over time.

PUBLIC HEALTH IMPLICATIONS

Findings from the current study demonstrate that methamphetamine-related mortality has increased dramatically over the last 2 decades, with the greatest annual increases occurring from 2014 to 2021. Moreover, an increasing proportion of these methamphetamine deaths co-involved heroin or fentanyl over time, with the greatest annual increases occurring from 2010 to 2021. Our results show that both the age-adjusted methamphetamine mortality rate and co-involvement of heroin or fentanyl were the greatest in 2021, with neither trend showing any sign of abatement. These findings underscore the need to develop, implement, and expand the availability and accessibility of robust harm reduction services, with particular attention to polysubstance use. AJPH

ABOUT THE AUTHORS

Rachel A. Hoopsick is with the Department of Kinesiology and Community Health, College of Applied Health Sciences, University of Illinois, Urbana-Champaign. R. Andrew Yockey is with the Department of Biostatistics and Epidemiology, University of North Texas Health Science Center, Fort Worth.

CORRESPONDENCE

Correspondence should be sent to Rachel A. Hoopsick, PhD, MS, MPH, MCHES, Department of Kinesiology and Community Health, College of Applied Health Sciences, University of Illinois Urbana-Champaign, 1206 S. Fourth St, 2017 Khan Annex, Huff Hall, Champaign, IL 61820 (e-mail: hoopsick@illinois.edu). Reprints can be ordered at http://www.ajph.org by clicking the "Reprints" link.

PUBLICATION INFORMATION

Full Citation: Hoopsick RA, Yockey RA. Methamphetamine-related mortality in the United States: co-involvement of heroin and fentanyl, 1999–2021. *Am J Public Health*. 2023;113(4): 416–419.

Acceptance Date: December 15, 2022.

DOI: https://doi.org/10.2105/AJPH.2022.307212

CONTRIBUTORS

R. A. Hoopsick conceptualized the study, conducted the statistical analyses, and wrote the first draft of the manuscript with sections contributed by R. A. Yockey. Both authors reviewed and approved the final version of this manuscript.

CONFLICTS OF INTEREST

The authors have no conflicts of interest to disclose.

HUMAN PARTICIPANT PROTECTION

The University of Illinois Urbana-Champaign institutional review board determined that this study was exempt from review.

REFERENCES

1. Friedman J, Akre S. COVID-19 and the drug overdose crisis: uncovering the deadliest months in the United States, January–July 2020. *Am J Public Health*. 2021;111(7):1284–1291. https://doi.org/10.2105/AJPH.2021.306256
2. National Center for Health Statistics. Drug overdose deaths in the US top 100,000 annually. 2021. Available at: https://www.cdc.gov/nchs/pressroom/nchs_press_releases/2021/20211117.htm. Accessed October 6, 2022.
3. Han B, Compton WM, Jones CM, Einstein EB, Volkow ND. Methamphetamine use, methamphetamine use disorder, and associated overdose deaths among US adults. *JAMA Psychiatry*. 2021;78(12):1329–1342. https://doi.org/10.1001/jamapsychiatry.2021.2588
4. Strickland JC, Stoops WW, Dunn KE, Smith KE, Havens JR. The continued rise of methamphetamine use among people who use heroin in the United States. *Drug Alcohol Depend*. 2021;225: 108750. https://doi.org/10.1016/j.drugalcdep.2021.108750
5. Hedegaard H, Miniño A, Warner M. Co-involvement of opioids in drug overdose deaths involving cocaine and psychostimulants. April 2021. NCHS Data Brief no. 406. https://doi.org/10.15620/cdc:103966
6. Ivsins A, Fleming T, Barker A, et al. The practice and embodiment of "goofballs": a qualitative study exploring the co-injection of methamphetamines and opioids. *Int J Drug Policy*. 2022; 107:103791. https://doi.org/10.1016/j.drugpo.2022.103791
7. Mansoor M, McNeil R, Fleming T, et al. Characterizing stimulant overdose: a qualitative study on perceptions and experiences of "overamping." *Int J Drug Policy*. 2022;102:103592. https://doi.org/10.1016/j.drugpo.2022.103592
8. Park JN, Rashidi E, Foti K, Zoorob M, Sherman S, Alexander GC. Fentanyl and fentanyl analogs in the illicit stimulant supply: results from US drug seizure data, 2011–2016. *Drug Alcohol Depend*. 2021;218:108416. https://doi.org/10.1016/j.drugalcdep.2020.108416
9. DiGennaro C, Garcia G-GP, Stringfellow EJ, Wakeman S, Jalali MS. Changes in characteristics of drug overdose death trends during the COVID-19 pandemic. *Int J Drug Policy*. 2021;98:103392. https://doi.org/10.1016/j.drugpo.2021.103392
10. Centers for Disease Control and Prevention, National Center for Health Statistics. CDC Wide-ranging ONline Data for Epidemiologic Research: multiple cause of death. Available at: https://wonder.cdc.gov. Accessed July 18. 2022.

Structural Racism and Pedestrian Safety: Measuring the Association Between Historical Redlining and Contemporary Pedestrian Fatalities Across the United States, 2010–2019

Nandi L. Taylor, MPH, Jamila M. Porter, DrPH, MPH, Shenee Bryan, MPH, MPA, Katherine J. Harmon, PhD, and Laura S. Sandt, PhD

See also Jacoby, p. 356.

AJPH April 2023, Vol 113, No. 4

Objectives. To examine the association between historical redlining and contemporary pedestrian fatalities across the United States.

Methods. We analyzed 2010–2019 traffic fatality data, obtained from the Fatality Analysis Reporting System, for all US pedestrian fatalities linked by location of crash to 1930s Home Owners' Loan Corporation (HOLC) grades and current sociodemographic factors at the census tract level. We applied generalized estimating equation models to assess the relationship between the count of pedestrian fatalities and redlining.

Results. In an adjusted multivariable analysis, tracts graded D ("Hazardous") had a 2.60 (95% confidence interval = 2.26, 2.99) incidence rate ratio (per residential population) of pedestrian fatalities compared with tracts graded A ("Best"). We found a significant dose–response relationship: as grades worsened from A to D, rates of pedestrian fatalities increased.

Conclusions. Historical redlining policy, initiated in the 1930s, has an impact on present-day transportation inequities in the United States.

Public Health Implications. To reduce transportation inequities, understanding how structurally racist policies, past and present, have an impact on community-level investments in transportation and health is crucial. (*Am J Public Health*. 2023;113(4):420–428. https://doi.org/10.2105/AJPH.2022.307192)

Transportation is an important social determinant of health that affects the ability of people to move efficiently and safely through public and private spaces. Active transportation—specifically walking, cycling, and rolling—has direct and indirect impacts on health at both individual and community levels.[1] Injuries and deaths among road users, especially those walking, continue to be a significant public health problem. In the past decade, pedestrian deaths have risen by 54% while all other traffic deaths have increased by 13%.[2] Low-income communities and communities of color bear a disproportionate burden of pedestrian injuries and fatalities, with Native/Indigenous and Black pedestrians being especially overrepresented.[3–8] Moreover, roadway designs that enable speeding and discourage walking are more likely to be in areas that experience high rates of pedestrian fatalities, which are often lower-income, Black, or Hispanic/Latinx communities.[9,10] However, research focuses on identifying factors that increase or decrease risk rather than characterizing the policies that created and facilitated these unsafe built environments.

There is a current shift in public health, both research and fields of practice, that seeks to understand the ways in which structural racism fundamentally causes the health inequities we see today in the United States. Bailey et al. define structural racism as

> the totality of ways in which societies foster racial discrimination, through mutually reinforcing inequitable systems (in housing, education, employment, earnings, benefits, credit, media, health care, criminal justice, and so on) that in turn reinforce discriminatory beliefs, values, and distribution of resources, which together affect the risk of adverse health outcomes.[11(p1454)]

Inequities in residential housing practices measured by residential racial segregation or historical redlining are a common indicator of structural racism.[12] "Redlining" is a term that refers to a federally sponsored policy that was initiated in the United States in the 1930s. The government-sponsored Home Owners' Loan Corporation (HOLC), created as part of President Franklin D. Roosevelt's New Deal, made loans to new homeowners by refinancing mortgages at low-interest rates. HOLC used color-coded and letter-graded maps to group neighborhoods into financial risk and lending categories.[13] Areas color-coded green ("A" or "Best") and blue ("B" or "Still Desirable") were predominantly White and were systematically approved for privately and publicly guaranteed home loans. However, neighborhoods color-coded yellow ("C" or "Definitely Declining") and red ("D" or "Hazardous"), which were populated by Black people and immigrants, were denied homeownership loans, ultimately impacting generational wealth and limiting community-level investments. Redlining legalized discrimination in housing and systematized structural racism on a national scale.[14] For an example of the language and maps created by HOLC, see Figure 1 and Figure A (available as a supplement to the online version of this article at https://ajph.org).[15]

Redlining is associated with a wide variety of contemporary adverse health outcomes, both at the individual and community level. These health outcomes include (but are not limited to) smoking, infant mortality, life expectancy, and firearm violence.[16–24] Krieger et al. found that census tracts assigned worse HOLC grades in New York City had an elevated risk of adverse maternal health outcomes.[19] Research on violence and historical redlining also found that neighborhoods that were redlined (graded D) in Louisville, Kentucky, had a greater incidence of gun violence compared with areas graded A, even after adjusting for census-level demographic factors.[16] Moreover, redlining continues to be associated with racial segregation, poverty, and income inequality.[23,25] Mitchell et al. found that areas graded "Hazardous" by redlining maps remain areas with lower household incomes.[25] By tying the presence of Black people to low property values, negating the generational wealth of Black households, cementing the racial wealth gap, and perpetuating disinvestment in segregated Black neighborhoods, redlining continues to adversely affect community health throughout the United States.

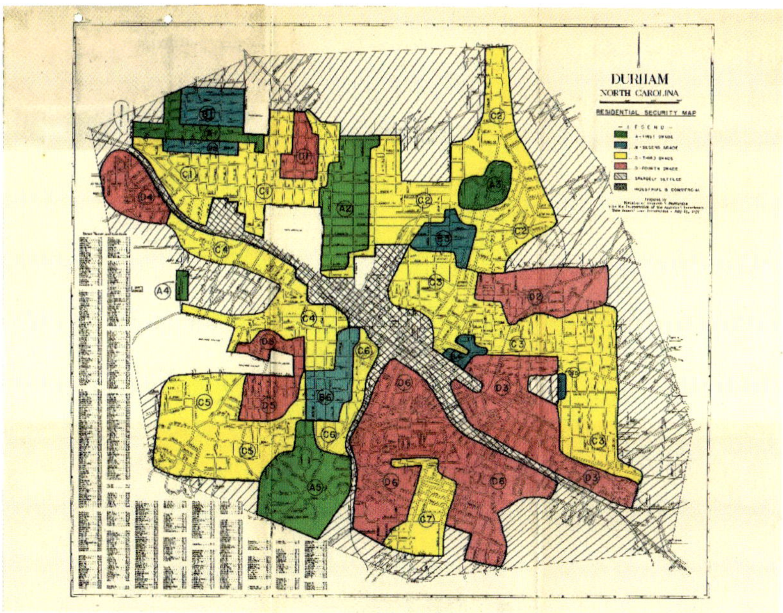

Color Code and Letter Grade	Description Example
A = "Best"	"Upward trend of desirability over the next 10–15 years."
B = "Still Desirable"	"A slow downward trend of desirability over the next 10–15 years."
C = "Definitely Declining"	"Downward trend of desirability over the next 10–15 years."
D = "Hazardous"	"Downward trend of desirability over the next 10–15 years."

FIGURE 1— 1930s Home Owners' Loan Corporation Map for Durham, North Carolina, and Grade-Related Descriptions: University of Richmond Mapping Inequality

Source. Nelson et al.[15]

To date, potential connections between redlining and transportation-related health outcomes have not been explored. Previous research has focused on how specific demographic, environmental, and behavioral factors are associated with pedestrian injuries and fatalities and may contribute to observed disparities in safety outcomes.[7,8,26] However, there is a gap in knowledge surrounding the impacts of inequitable neighborhood-level investments created by historical structurally racist policies, such as redlining and transportation-related disinvestments. As the field of traffic safety shifts from focusing primarily on changing individual-level factors to transforming structures that reinforce inequities in the transportation systems, there will be a need to understand how policies have created these inequitable systems. To hypothesize these relationships, we used a conceptual model to identify potential pathways between redlining and contemporary, neighborhood-level inequities in pedestrian fatalities.

We sought to address a gap in transportation safety research by assessing the impact of historical policies on contemporary pedestrian safety outcomes. In this study, we aimed to assess the impact of historical redlining on pedestrian fatalities within the United States between 2010 and 2019. Given that redlining is a leading contributing factor to economic disinvestment in neighborhoods, which may lead to a lack of pedestrian infrastructure in redlined neighborhoods, we hypothesized that historical redlining is associated with pedestrian fatalities throughout the United States. Specifically, we hypothesized that areas impacted by redlining or classified as "Definitely Declining" or "Hazardous" (graded C or D, respectively) will have higher contemporary rates of pedestrian fatalities. To our knowledge, this is the first study that seeks to describe the relationship between historical redlining and present-day transportation-related health outcomes on a national scale.

METHODS

We obtained the geocoded locations of all US traffic-related pedestrian fatalities from 2010 to 2019 from the Fatality Analysis Reporting System from the National Highway Traffic Safety Administration.[27] Of the 53 407 pedestrian fatalities that occurred between 2010 and 2019, we omitted 412 from the analysis because of unusable latitude and longitude values that were unreported, reported as unknown, or not available. We mapped the remaining 52 995 usable geographic coordinates by using ArcMap version 10.8 (ESRI, Redlands, CA). We then aggregated the counts of the pedestrian fatalities at the census tract level by using the 2019 US TIGER/Line Shapefiles.

Determining Redlined Areas

Our main exposure of interest was historical redlining, measured by the color-coded, A–D grades illustrated in the 1930s HOLC maps (Figure 1). For our analyses, we obtained shapefiles of all original HOLC maps from the University of Richmond Mapping Inequality project.[15] The original HOLC boundaries do not align spatially with current census tract boundaries. Like other studies, we used the area of overlap technique to assign HOLC grades to census tracts.[16,17,28] We overlayed redlining shapefiles with 2019 US census tracts to determine the number of intersections and areas of HOLC grades that fell within each census tract. We selected the HOLC grade with the largest area within the census tract boundary as the HOLC color-coded categorization for that census tract. We dropped tracts with less than 10% area overlap with HOLC grades or coded as "E" (uncharacterized) in the data set from the analysis. We completed all spatial processes in ArcMap version 10.8.

Covariates

We obtained covariates of interest including census tract–level self-reported race, ethnicity, age, gender, poverty, education, and population density from the 2010–2015 (5-year) American Community Survey (ACS), based on categories and descriptions developed by the US Census.[29] These variables included the percentage of non-Hispanic Black/African American, Hispanic/Latinx, male, those older than 18 years, those older than 65 years, those in poverty aged 18 years or older, and those older than 25 years with at least a high school degree or completion of general education development. We regrouped all variables, except for population density, into discrete "high" and "low" categories using mean and median distributions. We included population density as a continuous variable.

Statistical Analysis

We used descriptive statistics to assess the relationship between historical redlining, pedestrian fatalities, and sociodemographic factors at the census tract level. Our dependent variable was the count of pedestrian fatalities per census tract; therefore, we used models that account for count distributions and clustering at the census tract. We assessed generalized estimating equation regression, with log function and exchangeable correlation, to model the relationship between historical redlining and counts of pedestrian fatalities. We calculated incidence rate ratios (IRRs) with 95% confidence intervals (CIs) using population as an offset. Because of the potential clustering of pedestrian fatalities within our study area, we assessed residual spatial dependence among census tracts by using Moran's *I* statistic. We found that our model indicated a weak but significant spatial dependence (Moran's *I* statistic = 0.06; $P < .001$).

First, we modeled the unadjusted relationship between historical redlining and pedestrian fatalities using grade A as the referent. Second, we assessed multivariable models, using the goodness-of-fit statistic, by adjusting for census-tract level age, gender, and population density. We did not include all sociodemographic factors because of concerns that these factors may be mediators and could lead to overadjustment in our models.[30] To determine if redlining exhibited a dose–response effect for pedestrian fatalities across HOLC grades A to D, we performed the Kruskal–Wallis test for trends. We performed all statistical analyses with SAS version 9.4 (SAS Institute, Cary, NC).

RESULTS

We included a total of 15 289 census tracts in our analysis. We excluded census tracts with less than a 10% overlay with 1930s HOLC areas (n = 2412), with HOLC grade E (n = 10), and with zero population according to the 2015 ACS (n = 96). Our final sample included 13 377 census tracts across 38 states and 202 cities. Table 1 shows the characteristics of our study population. Within areas impacted by redlining, a total of 9631 pedestrian fatalities occurred between 2010 and 2019 with a maximum count of pedestrian fatalities per census tract of 17 (mean = 0.72; SD = 1.2). Roughly 45.1% of our 13 377 census tracts were graded C (n = 6037) followed by D (28.5%; n = 3816), B (20.0%; n = 2671), and A (6.3%; n = 853).

The overall rate of pedestrian fatalities was 2.0 per 100 000 person-years, with tracts assigned worse HOLC grades having higher pedestrian fatality rates per 100 000 person-years: A = 1.1; B = 1.6; C = 1.9; and D = 2.6. In addition, sociodemographic factors also varied by HOLC grades. Tracts graded D had a higher percentage of people of color (non-Hispanic Black and Hispanic/Latinx) and poverty compared with other tracts (Figure 2).

Comparison of Models and Multivariable Analysis

Table 2 illustrates the relationship between HOLC grades, demographic factors, and pedestrian fatalities. In our multivariable analysis, we found a significant relationship between historical redlining and contemporary pedestrian fatalities. In model 1, the unadjusted IRRs for HOLC grade D was 2.33 (95% CI = 2.03, 2.60) times the rate of pedestrian fatalities compared with grade A (Table 2, model 1). Tracts graded C (IRR = 1.71; 95% CI = 1.50, 1.96) or B (IRR = 1.38; 95% CI = 1.20, 1.60) were also associated with a higher IRR for pedestrian fatalities compared with tracts graded A. The estimated IRR from tracts

TABLE 1— Census Tract-Level Sociodemographic Characteristics and Count of Pedestrian Fatalities (n = 13 377): United States, 2010–2019

Characteristics	Mean	Median	Min	Max	SD	IQR
Outcome: pedestrian fatalities, no.	0.7	0.0	0.0	17	1.7	1.0
Covariates—sociodemographic factors[a]						
Non-Hispanic Black, %	26.2	10.7	0.0	100	31.2	38.8
Hispanic/Latinx, %	21.5	10.2	0.0	100	25.3	26.5
Male, %	48.5	48.4	0.0	100	4.7	5.1
Aged > 18 y, %	78.1	77.9	37.1	100	7.9	9.7
Aged > 65 y, %	12.3	11.5	0.0	100	5.9	7.2
Poverty, %	21.0	18.5	0.0	100	13.4	16.5
Education for those aged ≥ 25 y, %	26.2	27.2	0.0	100	11.4	18.9
Population density per 1000	6.5	3.1	0.0	93.3	9.0	5.6

Note. IQR = interquartile range. Education includes those aged ≥ 25 years with at least a high school degree or completion of general education development. Poverty includes those aged ≥ 18 years; federal poverty level according to the US Census.

[a]2010–2015 American Community Survey.[29]

graded D to those graded A showed a significant dose–response relationship (Kruskal–Wallis test: $P < .001$). After adjusting for census tract–level demographic factors, the relationship between HOLC grade designation and pedestrian fatalities remained. When compared with tracts graded A, census tracts graded D (IRR = 2.60; 95% CI = 2.26, 2.99), C (IRR = 1.84; 95% CI = 1.61, 2.11), or B (IRR = 1.49; 95% CI = 1.29, 1.72) were associated with higher incidence rates of pedestrian fatalities (Table 2, model 2).

DISCUSSION

In this novel study, we found a significant relationship between structural racism via historical redlining and contemporary, neighborhood-level inequities in pedestrian fatalities across the United States. More specifically, we found that census tracts graded D ("Hazardous") in the 1930s had an increased rate of present-day pedestrian fatalities compared with tracts graded A or "Best." In addition, we found a significant dose–response relationship from grades A to D, meaning that as grade color categorization worsened, pedestrian fatality rates increased. This finding adds to the current literature describing the impact of historical redlining on present-day neighborhood-level health inequities.[11,16–18,21,22] Similar to other studies, after adjustment for present-day demographic factors, the effect of redlining remained significant in tracts graded D, C, and B as compared with tracts graded A or "Best."[16,21,22]

While redlining is not a perfect or sole measure of structural racism, the long-lasting and intergenerational effects of this structurally racist policy are undeniable. Similar to other research, our study showed that census

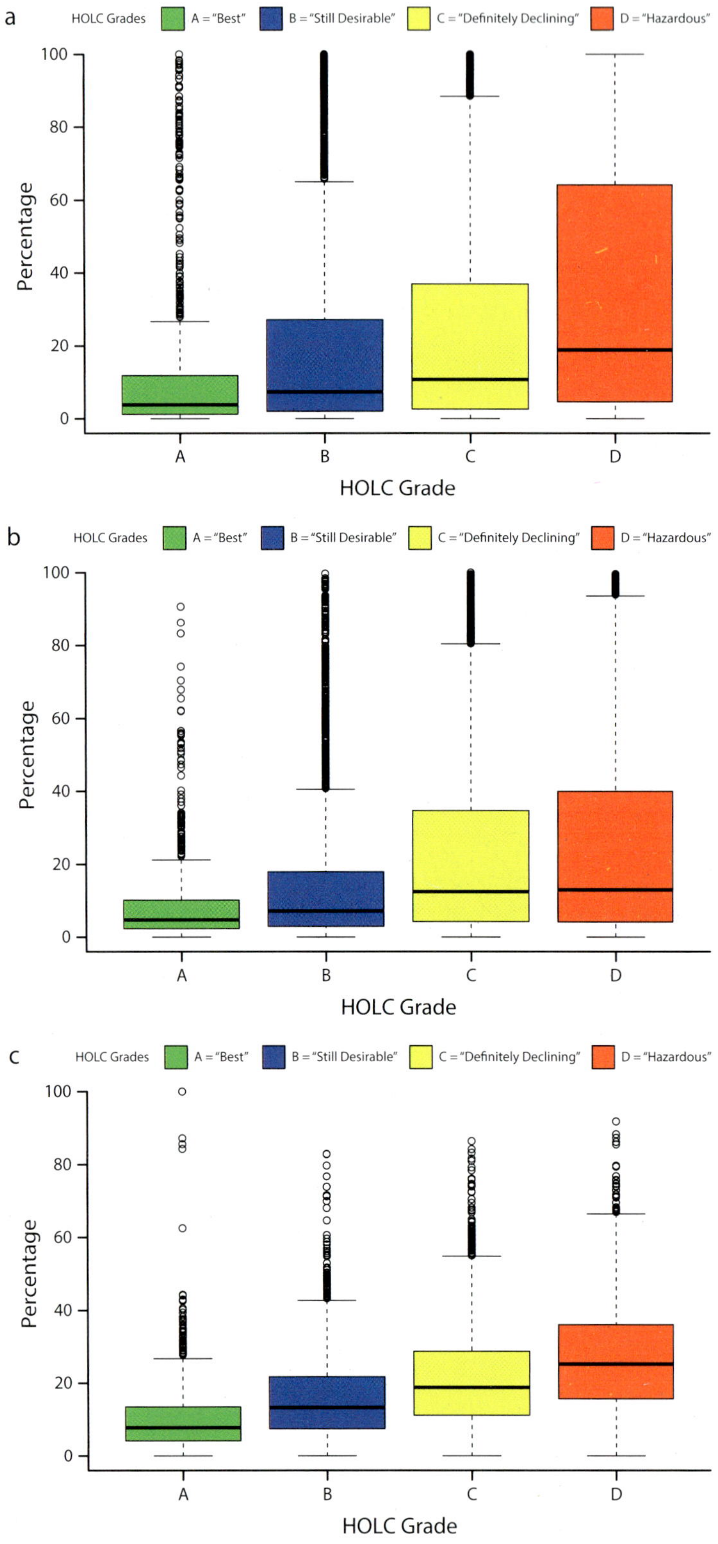

FIGURE 2— Census Tract-Level Characteristics by Home Owners' Loan Corporation (HOLC) Grade for (a) Non-Hispanic Black Persons, (b) Hispanic/Latinx Persons, and (c) Poverty: United States, 2010–2019

Note. Federal poverty level according to the US Census.
Source. 2010–2015 American Community Survey.[25]

TABLE 2— Multivariable Associations of Pedestrian Fatalities With Historical Redlining, Census Tract–Level Demographic Factors: Fatality Analysis Reporting System, United States, 2010–2019

	Model 1,[a] IRR (95% CI)	Model 2,[b] IRR (95% CI)	Model 3,[c] IRR (95% CI)
HOLC grade			
A (green)—"Best"	1 (Ref)	1 (Ref)	1 (Ref)
B (blue)—"Still Desirable"	1.38 (1.20, 1.60)	1.49 (1.29, 1.72)	1.49 (1.29, 1.72)
C (yellow)—"Definitely Declining"	1.71 (1.50, 1.96)	1.84 (1.61, 2.11)	1.84 (1.61, 2.11)
D (red)—"Hazardous"	2.33 (2.03, 2.68)	2.59 (2.25, 2.99)	2.60 (2.26, 2.99)
Model goodness of fit QIC[d]	2705.22	3077.49	3046.04

Note. CI = confidence interval; HOLC = Home Owners' Loan Corporation; IRR = incidence rate ratio; QIC = quasi likelihood under independence model criterion. Full descriptions of HOLC grades are in Figure A, available as a supplement to the online version of this article at https://ajph.org.

[a]Unadjusted, HOLC grade only.

[b]Fully adjusted for gender, age > 18 years, age > 65 years, and population density per 1000.

[c]Final model adjusted for age > 65 years and population density per 1000.

[d]The lowest goodness-of-fit statistic determines the best model.

tracts adversely impacted by historical redlining (graded D) continue to be areas with a higher percentage of populations that are impoverished and belong to communities of color.[25] Furthermore, research continues to show that areas with high poverty rates and reliance on public transit or active transportation (e.g., walking, rolling, and cycling) have an increased risk of pedestrian crashes and are often characterized by limited, unsafe, high-speed roadway infrastructure.[10,26]

Our findings indicate that redlining, a policy first implemented in the 1930s, which led to inequitable investments in communities, continues to adversely affect neighborhood-level transportation outcomes today. This is particularly noteworthy, given that most modern-day transportation safety programs, such as Vision Zero and the Safe System approach, do not typically acknowledge the impacts of structurally racist policies and racial inequities related to neighborhood-level transportation investments. They also do not undertake concrete efforts to rectify structural inequities in transportation and land use plans and investments. Rather than using "colorblind" approaches to transportation safety (e.g., allocating funds equally to communities for pedestrian infrastructure, regardless of the history of structural racism), these programs should aim to intentionally and directly address the underlying drivers of inequities in transportation safety and forge cross-agency partnerships with professionals in housing, community development, or public health to develop multidisciplinary approaches to rectify transportation inequities.

This study adds to a growing body of literature that confirms that historical policies that led to intergenerational neighborhood disinvestment must be redressed to improve public health, including the reduction of pedestrian fatalities throughout the nation. Departments of transportation at the local, state, and national level play key roles in the distribution and utilization of funding for roadway infrastructure, especially for large-scale highway projects. However, pedestrian infrastructure, such as sidewalks, is often left to the responsibility of private developers and property owners.[31] Therefore, lower-income neighborhoods often lack sidewalks or have poorly maintained sidewalks with limited connectivity. Structural racism has governed the trajectories of communities across the United States, creating multidecade place-based effects. These effects are often not acknowledged as a fundamental cause of transportation inequities. Individually focused behavioral countermeasures and siloed infrastructure projects cannot sufficiently address present-day inequities. Transportation researchers must understand and address upstream factors—like redlining—that continue to undermine positive population-level transportation outcomes.

To our knowledge, this is the first study that (1) connects redlining to transportation, a key social determinant of health, and (2) connects redlining to a transportation-related health outcome by collectively examining all known redlined cities across the United States. Contrasting with other studies that have focused on the identification of specific risk factors or countermeasures that might pertain to individual road users or roadway locations, this study focuses on root causes of inequities and quantifies the multigenerational effects on population-level health outcomes.

Research focused on the effects of historical redlining beyond a single or multicity level has been limited; however, our study examines the national-level impacts of historical redlining and neighborhood health. Our study underscores the ubiquity of this harmful policy and its longstanding effects on the health and safety of communities affected. Currently, the transportation and health communities suffer from an overreliance on individual-based research and behavior-based approaches to injury prevention, known to have limited effectiveness on complex, population-level challenges. More population-level research is needed to illuminate the effects of structural racism; assess historical, political, and social contexts; and highlight opportunities for systemic interventions that offer redress and high-impact, population-level health benefits.

Limitations

In our analysis, our outcome only included fatalities and did not include nonfatal injuries, which are also a significant public health problem. Although pedestrian fatalities are relatively rare events, census tracts with few or no fatalities may have had numerous nonfatal events. Moreover, residential population may not be the ideal denominator for examining exposure for all pedestrian behaviors (e.g., commuting or recreation); however, nationwide walking exposure information is limited. In addition, given that our data were aggregated to the census tract level, our findings are impacted by ecological fallacy. However, our findings support a well-established understanding that historical redlining impacts neighborhood-level health and can ultimately be used to explain place-based exposures and transportation inequities. Our results may also be impacted by both the uncertain geographic context problem and the modifiable areal unit problem. Census tracts are arbitrary boundaries, and pedestrian fatalities and roadway networks do not follow tract borders. However, less than 1% of crash locations fell within a 0.1-mile radius of borders that cross tracts that were graded D and A.

Our data are also subject to potential misclassification because of the assignment of 1930s HOLC grades to current-day census tracts when using overlay techniques. Roughly 16% of census tracts had less than 10% overlay with HOLC polygons, and removal of these tracts had little impact on our associations. While smaller geographic units may offer better resolution for interpretation of neighborhoods, studies using alternative geographic boundaries (e.g., HOLC polygons) have found similar results to our findings; therefore, we predict our relationship would remain.[17,24]

Furthermore, our analysis did not account for potential temporal changes in HOLC grades from the 1930s to the present day and did not measure changes to neighborhood-level trajectories in health and investment attributable to gentrification or displacement. However, like other studies, we found that redlined census tracts remain areas with higher percentages of populations that are impoverished and belong to communities of color.[16,19,23,25]

Despite controlling for census tract–level factors, there may still be unmeasured confounding effects, such as factors related to civic engagement, political power, or other processes that have an impact on policy decisions (e.g., voting rights). In addition, our analysis did not completely account for spatial dependence; therefore, to further address the relationship between historical redlining and transportation outcomes, studies should consider spatial analysis methods. Finally, our analysis focused on the national-level impacts of HOLC policies on present-day neighborhood-level pedestrian fatalities; therefore, findings cannot be used to determine the impacts of redlining on transportation safety within a specific city or state. Future studies may focus on smaller geographic areas to calibrate estimates and offer more context-specific interpretations.

Public Health Implications

Our study adds to the current literature by examining the legacy of structurally racist historical policies that perpetuated transportation inequities that can be observed today. Our study has a variety of implications for public health and transportation safety. Public health efforts that address traffic safety—such as Vision Zero and the Safe System approach—must focus on actions that modify the political, social, and built environments that result in inequitable transportation systems driven by structural racism. The US Department of Transportation Equity Action Plan identified equitable actions focused on empowering communities, expanding access, increasing resources, and wealth creation; however, more should be done to provide state and local guidance on best practices to measure and reduce inequities created by past and present policies and transportation investments including redlining.[32] Findings from this study underscore the importance of historical context and the availability of novel data sources, such as redlining maps, to support more nuanced and equity-focused decisions in land use, planning, policy-making, and transportation engineering.

Lessons learned from past interventions are also essential to public health approaches. Place-based funding interventions, often implemented by housing or revenue-focused governmental agencies, have increased property values and investment in disinvested communities; however, they have also led to gentrification and the residential displacement of low-income populations.[14,33] Some federal place-based funding programs that have attempted to equitably distribute funding to redlined areas have been associated with increases in property value.[14] However, these gains in neighborhood wealth were also associated with reductions in Black resident homeownership in areas formerly graded D.[14] These types of interventions show the possible benefits of place-based investments and reveal the consequences of displacement. Transportation interventions that focus on place-based funding should seek to reduce injuries and fatalities while also minimizing the consequences of displacement by centering community governance in transportation decision-making.

Future research should focus on 3 areas to address injury prevention inequities at the population level for pedestrian fatalities. First, more research is needed that focuses on measuring structural racism as the main exposure that drives health inequities. Racism is a public health crisis and has significant impacts on health across generations; however, investigations into how structural racism is a leading cause of transportation inequities have been limited and should be a focal point for future research. Analyzing other indicators of structural racism, such as school and residential racial segregation, racially discriminatory enforcement policies and practices, and the construction of high-speed roadways through communities of color, is important to understand and address present-day transportation inequities.[11,34]

Second, epidemiological research should focus on analyzing modifiable exposures, multidimensional pathways, and potential mediators that result in disparate outcomes for communities of color within the United States. Differences in specific built environment and roadway features, as well as impacts of gentrification and displacement, could be assessed in future studies to determine if relationships exist between the presence of these features, disinvestments tied to structurally racist policies like redlining, and present-day transportation outcomes.

Finally, research should focus on the intergenerational impacts of historical policies on neighborhood development that ultimately affect public health. Several pathways, at the community level—which include social, policy, and built environment factors—should be further explored to better understand how redlining is associated with pedestrian fatalities and to develop sustained policy solutions that focus on redress and make progress toward health and transportation equity. *AJPH*

ABOUT THE AUTHORS

Nandi L. Taylor is with the Injury Prevention Research Center and Department of Epidemiology, Gillings School of Global Public Health, University of North Carolina at Chapel Hill. Jamila M. Porter is with the Office of the CEO, de Beaumont Foundation, Bethesda, MD. Shenee Bryan is with S. Bryan Consulting LLC, Atlanta, GA. Katherine J. Harmon is with Injury Prevention Research Center and Highway Safety Research Center, University of North Carolina at Chapel Hill. Laura S. Sandt is with the Highway Safety Research Center, University of North Carolina at Chapel Hill.

CORRESPONDENCE

Correspondence should be sent to Nandi L. Taylor, MPH, UNC Injury Prevention Research Center and Department of Epidemiology, University of North Carolina at Chapel Hill, 725 Martin Luther King Jr Blvd, CB #7505, Chapel Hill, NC 27599 (e-mail: nandi.taylor@unc.edu). Reprints can be ordered at https://ajph.org by clicking the "Reprints" link.

PUBLICATION INFORMATION

Full Citation: Taylor NL, Porter JM, Bryan S, Harmon KJ, Sandt LS. Structural racism and pedestrian safety: measuring the association between historical redlining and contemporary pedestrian fatalities across the United States, 2010–2019. *Am J Public Health*. 2023;113(4):420–428.

Acceptance Date: November 23, 2022.

DOI: https://doi.org/10.2105/AJPH.2022.307192

CONTRIBUTORS

N. L. Taylor contributed to conceptualizing the study, conducted data management for geographic information system (GIS) processing of Home Owners' Loan Corporation (HOLC) grade and Fatality Analysis Reporting System (FARS) data, epidemiological methods, analysis, and interpretation of results, and led writing of the article. J. M. Porter conceptualized the study and contributed to writing and revising the article. S. Bryan contributed to conceptualizing the study, data management of FARS and HOLC data, and revision of the article. K. J. Harmon contributed to epidemiological methods, data analysis, interpretation of results, and revision of the article. L. S. Sandt contributed to the writing and revision of the article. All authors approved submission of the article to be published. We applied the sequence-determines-credit approach for the sequence of authors.

ACKNOWLEDGMENTS

This research was supported by the de Beaumont Foundation, a philanthropic organization dedicated to advancing policy, building partnerships, and strengthening public health, and the Collaborative Sciences Center for Road Safety, a US Department of Transportation National University Transportation Center promoting safety (USDOT grant 69A3551747113).

N. L. Taylor acknowledges William Covington for insights into GIS data management. N. L. Taylor and K. J. Harmon acknowledge Stephen W. Marshall, PhD, at the Injury Prevention Research Center at the University of North Carolina at Chapel Hill for insight into statistical analysis and methods.

Note. The contents of this study reflect the views of the authors, who are responsible for the facts and the accuracy of the information presented herein. This research is disseminated in the interest of information exchange. The study is funded, partially or entirely, by a grant from the US Department of Transportation's University Transportation Centers Program. However, the

US government assumes no liability for the contents or use thereof.

CONFLICTS OF INTEREST

All authors have no conflicts of interest to declare.

HUMAN PARTICIPANT PROTECTION

No protocol approval was needed for this study because the data used were publicly available, de-identified, and obtained from secondary sources.

REFERENCES

1. Office of Disease Prevention and Health Promotion, US Department of Health and Human Services. Social determinants of health. Healthy People 2030. Available at: https://health.gov/healthypeople. Accessed August 9, 2022.
2. Governors Highway Safety Association. Pedestrian traffic fatalities by state 2021 preliminary data. 2022. Available at: https://www.ghsa.org/resources/Pedestrians22. Accessed January 25, 2023.
3. Governors Highway Safety Association. An analysis of traffic fatalities by race and ethnicity. 2021. Available at: https://www.ghsa.org/resources/Analysis-of-Traffic-Fatalities-by-Race-and-Ethnicity21. Accessed June 29, 2022.
4. Chong SL, Chiang LW, Allen JC, Fleegler EW, Lee LK. Epidemiology of pedestrian–motor vehicle fatalities and injuries, 2006–2015. *Am J Prev Med.* 2018;55(1):98–105. https://doi.org/10.1016/j.amepre.2018.04.005
5. Harmon KJ, Peticolas K, Redding Erika M, Ising A, Waller AE. Examining the effect of pedestrian crashes on vulnerable populations in North Carolina. *N C Med J.* 2021;82(4):237–243. https://doi.org/10.18043/ncm.82.4.237
6. Hamann C, Peek-Asa C, Butcher B. Racial disparities in pedestrian-related injury hospitalizations in the United States. *BMC Public Health.* 2020;20(1):1459. https://doi.org/10.1186/s12889-020-09513-8
7. Sanders RL, Schneider RJ. An exploration of pedestrian fatalities by race in the United States. *Transp Res Part D Transp Environ.* 2022;107:103298. https://doi.org/10.1016/j.trd.2022.103298
8. Yu CY, Zhu X, Lee C. Income and racial disparity and the role of the built environment in pedestrian injuries. *J Plann Educ Res.* 2018;42(2):136–149. https://doi.org/10.1177/0739456X18807759
9. Lowe K. Environmental justice and pedestrianism: sidewalk continuity, race, and poverty in New Orleans, Louisiana. *Transp Res Rec.* 2016;2598(1):119–123. https://doi.org/10.3141/2598-14
10. Rajaee M, Echeverri B, Zuchowicz Z, Wiltfang K, Lucarelli JF. Socioeconomic and racial disparities of sidewalk quality in a traditional rust belt city. *SSM Popul Health.* 2021;16:100975. https://doi.org/10.1016/j.ssmph.2021.100975
11. Bailey ZD, Krieger N, Agénor M, Graves J, Linos N, Bassett MT. Structural racism and health inequities in the USA: evidence and interventions. *Lancet.* 2017;389(10077):1453–1463. https://doi.org/10.1016/S0140-6736(17)30569-X
12. Groos M, Wallace M, Hardeman R, Theall KP. Measuring inequity: a systematic review of methods used to quantify structural racism. *J Health Disparities Res Pract.* 2018;11(2):13. Available at: https://digitalscholarship.unlv.edu/jhdrp/vol11/iss2/13. Accessed February 13, 2023.
13. Hillier AE. Who received loans? Home Owners' Loan Corporation lending and discrimination in Philadelphia in the 1930s. *J Plann Hist.* 2003;2(1):3–24. https://doi.org/10.1177/1538513202239694
14. Robertson C, Parker E, Tach L. Historical redlining and contemporary federal place-based policy: a case of compensatory or compounding neighborhood inequality? *Hous Policy Debate.* 2022:1–24. https://doi.org/10.1080/10511482.2022.2026994
15. Nelson R, Winling L, Marciano R, et al. Mapping inequality. American Panorama. Available at: https://dsl.richmond.edu/panorama/redlining/#loc=4/36.71/-97.194. Accessed January 11, 2022.
16. Benns M, Ruther M, Nash N, Bozeman M, Harbrecht B, Miller K. The impact of historical racism on modern gun violence: redlining in the city of Louisville, KY. *Injury.* 2020;51(10):2192–2198. https://doi.org/10.1016/j.injury.2020.06.042
17. Huang SJ, Sehgal NJ. Association of historic redlining and present-day health in Baltimore. *PLoS ONE.* 2022;17(1):e0261028. https://doi.org/10.1371/journal.pone.0261028
18. Jacoby SF, Dong B, Beard JH, Wiebe DJ, Morrison CN. The enduring impact of historical and structural racism on urban violence in Philadelphia. *Soc Sci Med.* 2018;199:87–95. https://doi.org/10.1016/j.socscimed.2017.05.038
19. Krieger N, van Wye G, Huynh M, et al. Structural racism, historical redlining, and risk of preterm birth in New York City, 2013–2017. *Am J Public Health.* 2020;110(7):1046–1053. https://doi.org/10.2105/AJPH.2020.305656
20. Nardone A, Chiang J, Corburn J. Historic redlining and urban health today in US cities. *Environ Justice.* 2020;13(4):109–119. https://doi.org/10.1089/env.2020.0011
21. Poulson M, Neufeld MY, Dechert T, Allee L, Kenzik KM. Historic redlining, structural racism, and firearm violence: a structural equation modeling approach. *Lancet Reg Health Am.* 2021;3:100052. https://doi.org/10.1016/j.lana.2021.100052
22. Schwartz E, Onnen N, Craigmile PF, Roberts ME. The legacy of redlining: associations between historical neighborhood mapping and contemporary tobacco retailer density in Ohio. *Health Place.* 2021;68:102529. https://doi.org/10.1016/j.healthplace.2021.102529
23. Lynch EE, Malcoe LH, Laurent SE, Richardson J, Mitchell BC, Meier HCS. The legacy of structural racism: associations between historic redlining, current mortgage lending, and health. *SSM Popul Health.* 2021;14:100793. https://doi.org/10.1016/j.ssmph.2021.100793
24. Nardone A, Rudolph KE, Morello-Frosch R, Casey JA. Redlines and greenspace: the relationship between historical redlining and 2010 greenspace across the United States. *Environ Health Perspect.* 2021;129(1):17006. https://doi.org/10.1289/EHP7495
25. Mitchell B, Franco J. HOLC "redlining" maps: the persistent structure of segregation and economic inequality. 2018. Available at: https://dataspace.princeton.edu/bitstream/88435/dsp01dj52w776n/1/NCRC-Research-HOLC-10.pdf. Accessed June 10, 2022.
26. Lin PS, Guo R, Bialkowska-Jelinska E, Kourtellis A, Zhang Y. Development of countermeasures to effectively improve pedestrian safety in low-income areas. *J Traffic Transp Eng.* 2019;6(2):162–174. https://doi.org/10.1016/j.jtte.2019.02.001
27. National Highway Traffic Safety Administration. Fatality Analysis Reporting System. Available at: https://www.nhtsa.gov/file-downloads?p=nhtsa/downloads/FARS. Accessed November 17, 2021.
28. Noelke C, Outrich M, Baek M, et al. Connecting past to present: examining different approaches to linking historical redlining to present day health inequities. *PLoS One.* 2022;17(5):e0267606. https://doi.org/10.1371/journal.pone.0267606
29. US Census Bureau. American Community Survey. Available at: https://www.census.gov/programs-surveys/acs. Accessed March 3, 2022.
30. Schisterman EF, Cole SR, Platt RW. Overadjustment bias and unnecessary adjustment in epidemiologic studies. *Epidemiology.* 2009;20(4):488–495. https://doi.org/10.1097/EDE.0b013e3181a819a1
31. Gelinne D. Steps to prioritize and implement sidewalks. *Georgia's Cities Newspaper.* February 11, 2019. Available at: https://www.gacities.com/News/Viewpoints/Steps-to-Prioritize-and-Implement-Sidewalks.aspx. Accessed August 9, 2022.
32. US Department of Transportation. Equity Action Plan. 2022. Available at: https://www.transportation.gov/sites/dot.gov/files/2022-04/Equity_Action_Plan.pdf. Accessed July 27, 2022.
33. Marcuse P. Gentrification, abandonment, and displacement: connections, causes, and policy responses in New York City. *Wash U J Urb Contemp L.* 1985;28(1):195. Available at: https://openscholarship.wustl.edu/law_urbanlaw/vol28/iss1/4. Accessed July 6, 2022.
34. Hardeman RR, Homan PA, Chantarat T, Davis BA, Brown TH. Improving the measurement of structural racism to achieve antiracist health policy. *Health Aff (Millwood).* 2022;41(2):179–186. https://doi.org/10.1377/hlthaff.2021.01489.

Abortion-Related Laws and Concurrent Patterns in Abortion Incidence in Indiana, 2010–2019

Heidi Moseson, PhD, MPH, Mikaela H. Smith, PhD, Payal Chakraborty, PhD, MS, Hillary J. Gyuras, MA, Abigail Foster, BS, Danielle Bessett, PhD, Tracey A. Wilkinson, MD, MPH, and Alison H. Norris, MD, PhD

Objectives. To analyze abortion incidence in Indiana concurrent with changes in abortion-related laws.

Methods. Using publicly available data, we created a timeline of abortion-related laws in Indiana, calculated abortion rates by geography, and described changes in abortion occurrence coincident with changes in abortion-related laws between 2010 and 2019.

Results. Between 2010 and 2019, Indiana's legislature passed 14 abortion-restricting laws, and 4 of 10 abortion-providing clinics closed. The Indiana abortion rate decreased from 7.8 abortions per 1000 women aged 15 to 44 years in 2010 to 5.9 in 2019. At all time points, the abortion rate was 58% to 71% of the Midwestern rate and 48% to 55% of the national rate. By 2019, nearly 1 in 3 (29%) Indiana residents who obtained abortion care did so outside the state.

Conclusions. Access to abortion in Indiana over the past decade was low, required increases in interstate travel to obtain care, and co-occurred with the passage of numerous abortion restrictions.

Public Health Implications. These findings preview unequal abortion access and increases in interstate travel as state-level restrictions and bans go into effect across the country. (*Am J Public Health*. 2023;113(4):429–437. https://doi.org/10.2105/AJPH.2022.307196)

AJPH April 2023, Vol 113, No. 4

The United States has experienced a surge in abortion-related legislation over the past decade,[1] culminating in the overturning of federal protections for abortion by the US Supreme Court's *Dobbs v Jackson Women's Health Organization* opinion in June 2022.[2] In the 12 years leading up to the *Dobbs* opinion, states passed more than 470 state-level abortion restrictions that limited abortion access in direct (e.g., requiring unnecessary hospital admitting privileges)[3] and indirect (e.g., medically unnecessary waiting periods that can cause increases in travel)[4] ways and approximately 70 policies that protected abortion access.[5]

Compared with other state governments, Indiana's government has a particularly hostile legislative and policy history toward abortion[6]: the state enacted more abortion restrictions between 1973 and 2020 than most other states[7] and has consistently been categorized as very hostile toward abortion.[6] Restrictions have included an 18-hour waiting period following state-directed counseling, written and notarized parental consent or judicial bypass requirements for minors, prohibition on the use of telemedicine to administer medication abortion, limitations on abortion provision beyond 14 weeks gestation, and severe restrictions on public funding for abortion.[8] With the removal of constitutional protections for abortion, however, Indiana became the first state in the country to pass a ban on abortion at zero weeks and immediate delicensure of all freestanding abortion clinics.[9] The law went into effect on September 15, 2022, with limited exceptions for rape and incest (up to 12 weeks of pregnancy dated from last menstrual period), fatal fetal diagnoses (up to 22 weeks after last menstrual period), and the life and health of the pregnant person. One week later, a judge granted a preliminary injunction on the ban. On October 12, 2022, the Indiana Supreme Court allowed the injunction to stand and abortions to continue at least until a ruling is issued following oral arguments that took place on January 19, 2023—typically issued at least 2 months after the hearing.

Counter to their stated intention of protecting pregnant people's health, laws restricting abortion access have been demonstrated to increase mortality and morbidity during pregnancy,[10] to delay or block access to necessary health care, and to otherwise burden or harm abortion seekers and providers.[3,11] But abortion care access is not just a critical component of public health, it is also essential to reproductive autonomy and justice.[12] At its core, abortion access recognizes each individuals' fundamental right to bodily autonomy, and the repercussions of granting versus denying that right are profound. Among the many established benefits of abortion access are improved physical health,[13] lower risk of intimate partner violence,[14] improved socioeconomic conditions,[15] and better developmental outcomes for one's existing and subsequent children.[16]

Given its history of abortion restrictions, Indiana can serve as a case study for examining how changes in abortion policy coincide with changes in abortion utilization, especially as more states enact extremely restrictive abortion bans—including total abortion bans and bans after the detection of fetal cardiac activity—following the loss of federal abortion protections. The demographic makeup of the state allows some examination of how abortion restrictions may affect abortion seekers unevenly in terms of geography: Indiana's 92 counties are almost equally split between metropolitan (44) and nonmetropolitan (48).[17,18]

However, the peer-reviewed research on abortion incidence or abortion care–seeking experiences in Indiana is extremely scarce. A 1997 study examined the impact of parental involvement laws on abortion incidence among minors in Indiana and found that these laws reduced the in-state abortion rate for minors, delayed them in obtaining abortion care, and increased their out-of-state travel.[19] Aside from this 1997 study, we identified no peer-reviewed public health research on abortion access in Indiana. To address this gap in the literature, we endeavored to provide a descriptive review of Indiana's regulatory environment over the past decade and to conduct an empirical analysis of abortion incidence patterns in the state. We evaluated abortion incidence overall and by duration of pregnancy in the state versus in the region and in the nation. We also determined abortion incidence by Indiana county as well as Indiana residents' out-of-state abortion utilization between 2010 and 2019, the most recent years for which data are available.

METHODS

Data on individual abortion-related laws, including dates of proposal and enactment, were from the Indiana General Assembly Web site, supplemented by researcher review of news reports, court filings, and legal advocacy organization reports. Specifically, we used the search by subject function on the Indiana General Assembly Web site to locate each piece of abortion-related legislation signed into law between 2014 and 2019, and we then reviewed the Indiana General Assembly's list of archived bills to locate those related to abortion between 2010 and 2013. We cross-referenced the list of legislation with Indiana abortion laws included in the LawAtlas (https://lawatlas.org) and Guttmacher Institute Web sites. From these sources, we extracted and organized information on abortion-related laws in Indiana into a table, including content and dates of enactment. Using this compiled data set, we then created a timeline that depicts Indiana's new abortion-related laws over the past decade and plotted these alongside concurrent abortion-providing clinic closures and openings.

Data on the number and location of sites providing abortions in Indiana were from Indiana Department of Health Clinical Licensing Program materials (publicly available on the Indiana Department of Health Web site between 2008 and 2020) as well as from newspaper articles, court records, and digital archives (via the Wayback Machine). From these data, we determined the number of abortion facilities in the state for each year. We used this to calculate the facility density (i.e., facilities per million women aged 15–44 years) by extracting the number of facilities in the state from the Indiana State Licensing program data and dividing this by the US Census estimate of the number of women aged 15 to 44 years in the state for that year. We similarly estimated facility density for the Midwest and the United States, extracting data on the number of facilities from Guttmacher Institute data[20]; however, because Guttmacher Institute data on facility numbers are available only for 2014 and 2017, we calculated facility density for the Midwest and the United States for these 2 years only. We used the word "women" in our description of denominators to be consistent with the language of the US Census methods that generated these estimates, but we acknowledge that this is a limitation of the measure because transgender, nonbinary, and gender-expansive people also have abortions.

Measures

To calculate abortion rates (number of abortions per year per 1000 women aged 15–44 years) over time by county, state, region, the United States, and percentage of patients leaving their state of residence for abortion care, we accessed several publicly available state- and national-level data sets. Publicly available data included Centers for Disease Control and Prevention (CDC) annual abortion surveillance reports,[21] Indiana Department of Health Terminated Pregnancy Reports,[22] and the US Census.[23] To calculate the abortion rate in Indiana, we extracted the number of abortions that took place in Indiana (abortions by occurrence) for each year between 2010 and 2019 from CDC data and divided this by the US Census estimate of the number of women aged 15 to 44 years in Indiana for that year.

To calculate the abortion rate in the Midwestern region, we similarly extracted the number of abortions that took place in all states with a Midwestern designation in the US Census (IL, IN, IA, KS, MI, MN, MO, NE, ND, OH, SD, and WI) and divided this annual total of Midwestern abortions by the US Census estimate of the number of women aged 15 to 44 years in those 12 states for each year. Finally, to calculate the national abortion rate, we extracted the total number of abortions reported in the United States for each year and divided each annual abortion total by the US Census estimate for the number of women aged 15 to 44 years in the states that reported abortions in that year.

Because reporting data to the CDC is voluntary, not all states report abortion counts to the CDC and thus are missing from the CDC estimates. Specifically, we excluded the following states when calculating national abortion rates because of either not reporting to the CDC or not following reporting guidelines: California, Maryland, New Hampshire, and New Jersey (2010–2019); District of Columbia and Wyoming (2010–2018); Maine (2012); and Florida (2010–2016, for rates by residence only).

To create abortion rates for each county in Indiana, we extracted the total number of abortions reported for each county in each year from the Terminated Pregnancy Reports data and divided that by the US Census data's estimated number of women aged 15 to 44 years in each county. To explore abortion rates by county classification (metro, urban, or rural), we relied on a county classification system based on the US Department of Agriculture rural–urban continuum codes, most recently updated in 2013.[17] Specifically, the Department of Agriculture designates counties as "metro" (based on Office of Management and Budget metro designations[24]), "nonmetro–urban" (nonmetro and ≥ 2500 people), and "nonmetro–rural" (nonmetro and < 2500 people). The Indiana Termination of Pregnancy Reports designated counties that saw between 1 and 5 abortions per year as missing; to include these 10 counties in the analysis, we assigned them as having 3 abortions each (the median value in the possible range).

To calculate the percentage of Indiana residents who left the state to obtain an abortion, we extracted the number of abortions Indiana residents obtained out of state each year from the CDC surveillance reports and divided this out-of-state abortion count by the total number of abortions that Indiana residents received (inside and outside the state) for that year, per Smith et al.[25] For Midwest and national estimates, we repeated the steps using counts for each specific region. We excluded all states that were missing or had incomplete data from any of our study years to keep consistent the states represented across years. To examine the states to which Indiana residents traveled to obtain their abortions, we used the same CDC data to obtain the total number of abortions Indiana residents received each year in each of the states that reported abortions given to Indiana residents for each year between 2010 and 2019.

Data Analysis

To evaluate patterns in abortion rate over the full period, we calculated percentage changes in abortion rates as follows: $(rate_{2019} - rate_{2010})/rate_{2010}$. To calculate average abortion rates for metro, urban, and rural counties, we summed county-level rates for all counties with the specific classification and divided by the number of counties with that designation. To present findings visually, we plotted key results over time via line graphs or maps.

We used Stata version 17 (StataCorp, College Station, TX) for all analyses and ArcGIS Pro (Esri, Redlands, CA) for all maps.

RESULTS

Between 2010 and 2019, Indiana's state legislature passed 14 abortion-restricting bills; all contained multiple provisions (Table A, available as a supplement to the online version of this article at http://www.ajph.org). Although each bill was signed into law by the governor, 6 were blocked from going into effect—in whole or in part—because of court cases challenging their constitutionality. Those that went into effect included requirements for abortion providers to have written admitting privileges at nearby hospitals (i.e., formal agreements between a physician and a specific hospital allowing the physician to directly admit patients to the hospital and provide services to their patients in that hospital as medical staff), restrictions on judicial bypass options for minors, and a telemedicine ban.

Abortion-Providing Facilities

During this period, shifts occurred in the number of abortion-providing facilities in Indiana (Figure 1). In 2010, there were 9 clinics that provided procedural abortions and 1 additional clinic that provided only medication abortion services. Between 2010 and 2019, 4 of these 10 abortion-providing clinics closed and 1 new clinic opened in 2019, so that Indiana had a facility density of 7.7 in 2010 and 5.4 in 2019. The densities are slightly lower than are those in the Midwest (7.4 in 2014 and 7.0 in 2017) and less than half those in the United States (15.3 in 2014 and 15.5 in 2017).

Abortion Incidence

The abortion rate by state of provision in Indiana decreased from 7.8 abortions per 1000 women aged 15 to 44 years in 2010 to 5.9 abortions in 2019 (Table B, part 1, available as a supplement to the online version of this article at http://www.ajph.org; Figure 2a). Although the United States and the Midwestern regions also saw a decline in the abortion rate by state of provision over this period, the decline in the abortion rate in Indiana (24%) was more than 3 times that of the decrease in the Midwest region (7%) and slightly more than the decrease in the United States (20%). Notably, the in-state Indiana abortion rate is lower than are the regional and national rates throughout this period; in any given year, the Indiana abortion rate by state of provision was only 48% to 55% of the national abortion rate and 58% to 71% of the Midwestern rate.

Conversely, the abortion rate by state of residence did not decrease as sharply over the same period (Table B, part 2; Figure 2b). The abortion rate among Indiana residents, including Indiana residents who traveled out of state for their abortions, decreased by 11%—only 46% of the decrease seen in the abortion rate in Indiana and like the decrease observed nationally (10%). Thus, the abortion rate among Indiana

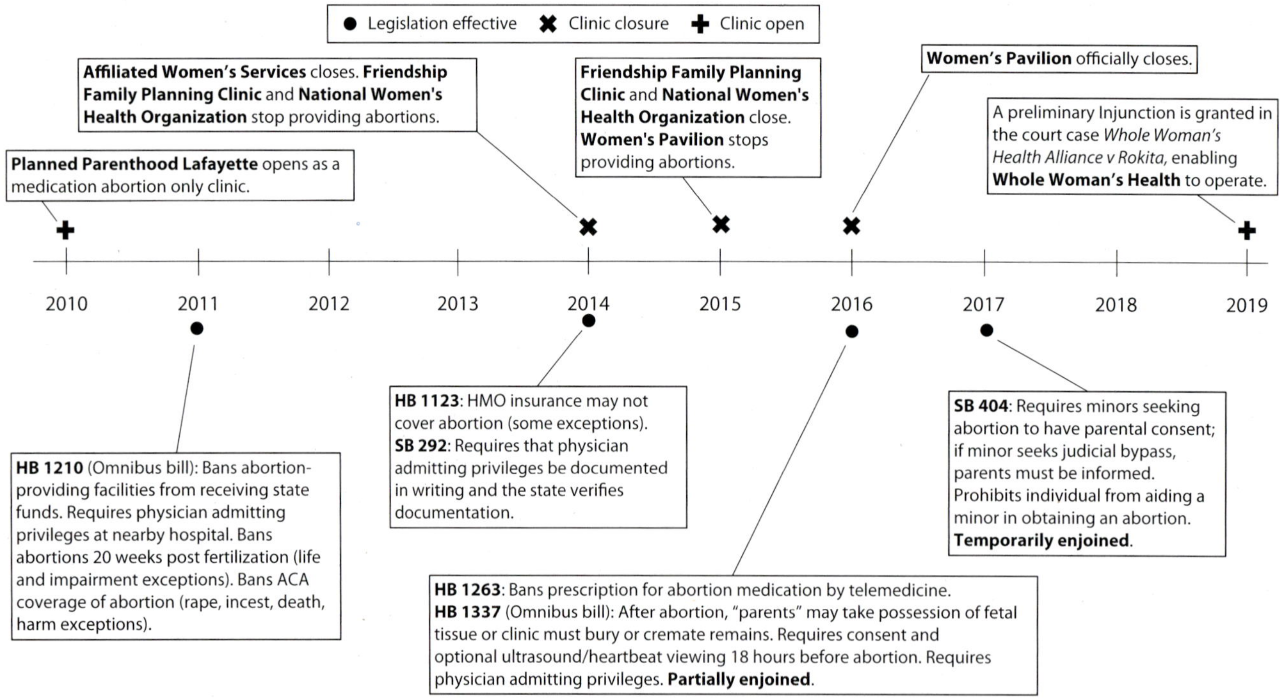

FIGURE 1— Abortion-Related Legislation and Facility Closures in Indiana: 2010–2019

Note. ACA = Affordable Care Act; HMO = health maintenance organization.

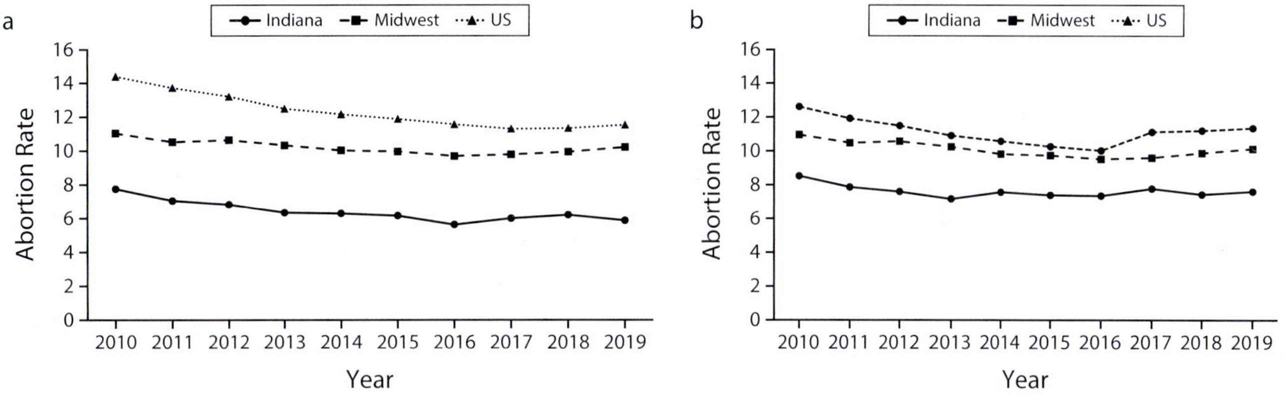

FIGURE 2— Abortion Rate (Abortions per 1000 Women Aged 15–44 Years) in Indiana, the Midwest, and the United States by (a) State of Provision, and (b) State of Residence: 2010–2019

Note. Midwestern states include IL, IN, IA, KS, MI, MN, MO, NE, ND, OH, SD, and WI. We excluded the following states in national totals for the following years: CA, MD, NH, and NJ (2010–2019); DC and WY (2010–2018); ME (2012); and FL (2010–2016 for rates by residence).

residents did not decrease as steeply as the abortion rate within the borders of the state.

Abortions by County

The average abortion rate from 2010 to 2019 was highest among people from Indiana's metropolitan counties (6.7 per 1000 women aged 15–44 years), followed by those from urban, nonmetropolitan counties (3.1 per 1000 women aged 15–44 years) and then by rural, nonmetropolitan counties (1.5 per 1000 women aged 15–44 years; Figure 3). The metropolitan rate has decreased over time, whereas the urban and rural rates have remained extremely low. When comparing abortion rates and facility locations in 2010 versus 2019 (Figure 3), decreases in rates in the northwest corner of the state are particularly notable given the loss of a clinic there between 2010 and 2019.

Out-of-State Travel for Abortion Care

Both the number and percentage of Indiana residents traveling out of state for abortion care ("percentage leaving") increased between 2010 and 2019: from 13% of all abortions (1471) in 2010 to 29% (2868) in 2019 (Table C, available as a supplement to the online version of this article at http://www.ajph.org; Figure 4). Compared with the region and the United States, Indiana has a higher average percentage leaving over the 10-year period (22% vs 9% in the Midwest and 7% nationally), and Indiana's percentage leaving more than doubled over the period, whereas national and Midwest percentages leaving increased only slightly.

Indiana residents who left the state for abortion care between 2010 and 2019 traveled to 1 of 4 states: Illinois, Kentucky, Michigan, or Ohio (Figure A, available as a supplement to the online version of this article at https://www.ajph.org). From 2011 through 2019, an increasing majority of those who traveled for abortion care went to neighboring Illinois, a state with fewer abortion restrictions.[1]

DISCUSSION

This retrospective analysis of abortion-related laws and abortion incidence in Indiana between 2010 and 2019 highlights that (1) abortion utilization was strikingly lower in Indiana than the region and the nation, (2) abortion utilization was unequal across the state, and (3) a high and increasing proportion of Indiana residents traveled outside the state for abortion care. With abortion incidence in Indiana consistently lower than that in Midwestern regional levels, and with nearly 1 in 3 patients who had abortions leaving the state to obtain abortion care, Indiana residents did not have sufficient abortion care access in their home state—even before the enactment of the full abortion ban in September 2022 and the legal uncertainty following injunction.

Study findings demonstrate inequities in abortion access in Indiana by geography. Residents in rural counties had an extremely low abortion rate over the period analyzed—only 22% of the abortion rate of Indiana residents who lived in metropolitan counties. This pattern is similar to that observed in neighboring Ohio, where abortion is also accessed more frequently by people living in urban areas and least by people living in rural areas.[26] This may be the result of

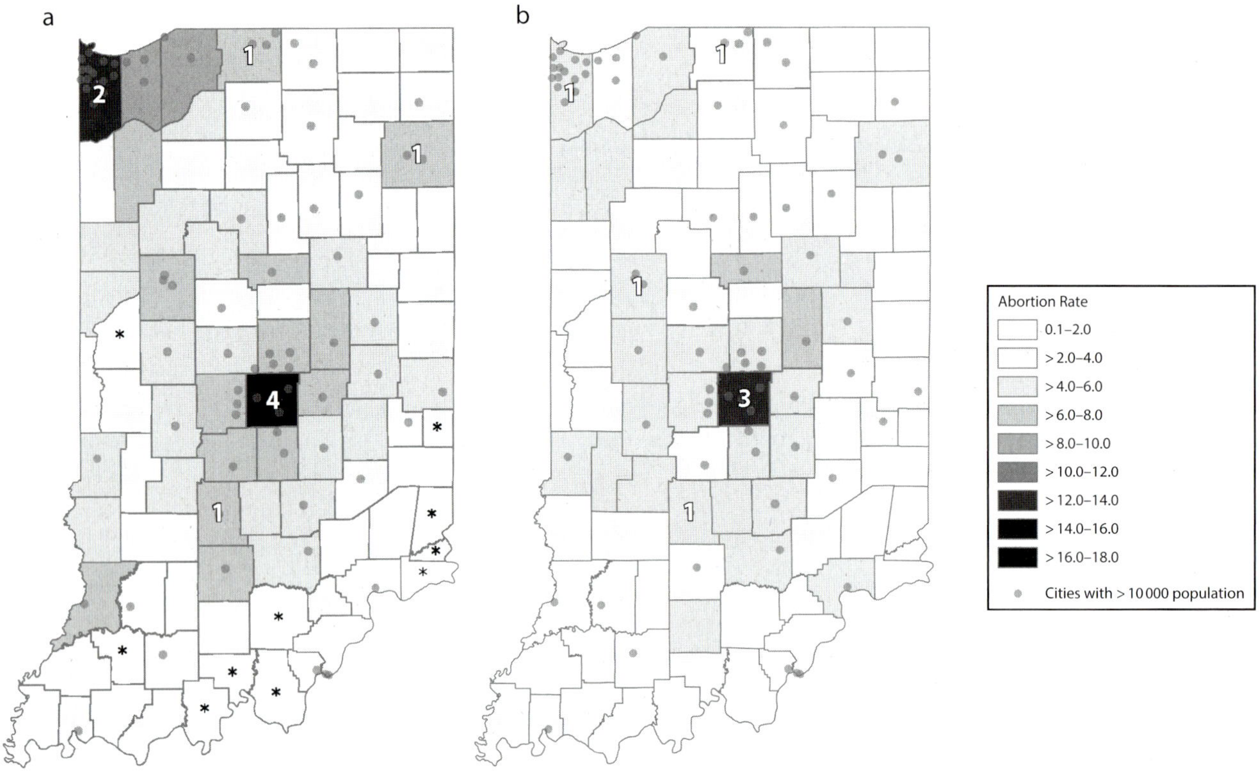

FIGURE 3— Abortion Rate by County of Residence (Abortions per 1000 Indiana Women Aged 15–44 Years) and Number of Abortion Clinics in the County in (a) 2010 and (b) 2019

*Ten counties (Crawford, Dearborn, Fountain, Harrison, Ohio, Perry, Pike, Switzerland, Union, and Washington) had between 1 and 5 patients who had abortions; rates included here are based on the median of 3 patients for these counties.

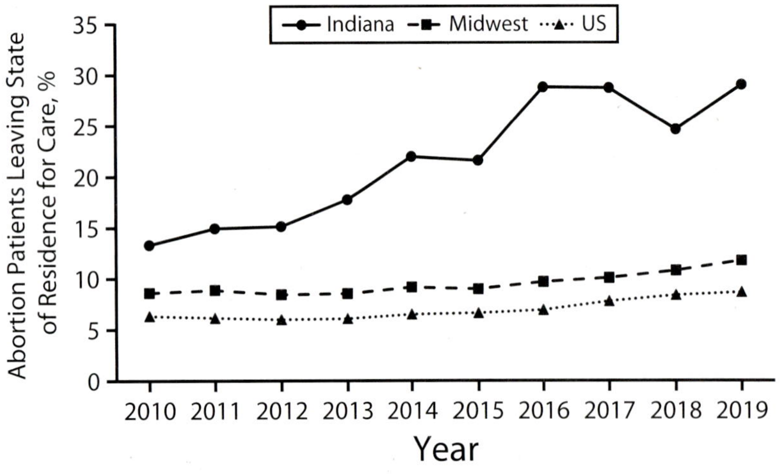

FIGURE 4— Percentage of Patients Who Had Abortions Leaving Their State of Residence for the Abortion: Comparing Residents in Indiana, the Midwest, and the United States: 2010–2019

a larger trend of reproductive health access deserts in rural areas[27–29] and could be exacerbated by Indiana laws that require abortion providers to have admitting privileges at nearby hospitals, thereby restricting abortion-providing facilities to being located primarily in urban areas near hospitals.[3]

Furthermore, these findings reveal a high and increasing percentage of Indiana residents who left the state to access abortion care. People seeking abortion care may travel out of their state of residence for many reasons, including policy-driven requirements related to gestational limits,[29] waiting periods,[30] parental notification, and judicial bypass[31] or simply location convenience (i.e., the closest clinic to them is in another state)[32] or shorter wait times.[33] Our finding that the percentage of people leaving Indiana for abortion care increased sharply from 13% to 29% alongside a decade of policy restrictions and facility closures reflects a larger US trend in which states with more restrictive abortion laws or a lower facility density have a higher percentage of patients leaving the state for care.[25] Although the rate of abortions taking place in Indiana decreased across our study period, the rate among people from Indiana was relatively consistent, reflecting a continued need for abortions among Indiana residents and thus the increasing percentage of those leaving over time.

Given the legal uncertainty following the total abortion ban enacted and enjoined in September 2022, the number of Indiana residents who will need support to travel across state lines to access abortion care in Illinois or another state may increase dramatically.[34] Previous research indicates that burdens associated with interstate travel include lack of insurance coverage as well as additional costs associated with transportation, overnight stays, missing work, and childcare.[25] Given that nearly one third of Indiana abortion recipients in 2019 were already traveling out of state for care and that there was an anticipated increase in this percentage following uncertainty induced by Indiana's contested abortion ban, the financial and logistical support that Indiana residents will need to obtain abortion care will correspondingly increase. Importantly, these burdens associated with increased travel are likely experienced disproportionately. Particularly affected are Black people, Indigenous people, and other people of color; transgender and nonbinary people; and those experiencing financial hardships. This is true especially given racism in the reproductive health care system[35–38] as well as experiences of reproductive oppression and coercion on the pathway to abortion care.[39,40] Targeted outreach and support for abortion seekers from these communities will be an important public health imperative.

Limitations and Strengths

Although these findings highlight important aspects of abortion access in Indiana, we note that these aggregate data do not provide information on individual experiences, particularly barriers or facilitators to abortion access in the state. Although we see aggregate differences in abortion incidence by geography, our data cannot speak to the overlapping barriers that Indiana residents may face when seeking reproductive health care, particularly for adolescents, those with marginalized racial or gender identities, and those who are struggling financially.[41] Future work should examine how systems of racial oppression intersect with class- and location-based forms of oppression to result in differential access to care. Our data also cannot illuminate the experience of people who wanted abortions and were unable to obtain one in Indiana or in a neighboring state, and yet certainly there are people unrepresented in our findings for whom the barriers were insurmountable.[42]

Furthermore, because of missingness in CDC data from several key states that do not routinely provide data on abortion incidence to the CDC, we likely underestimated the national abortion rate in this analysis. Therefore, our comparison of the Indiana abortion rate to the national abortion rate likely underestimates the magnitude of the difference between Indiana's trends and national trends and thereby underestimates how much lower abortion access is in Indiana than nationally. This is a conservative bias and is quantified in Table D (available as a supplement to the online version of this article at http://www.ajph.org), which presents the CDC and Guttmacher rates side by side for the years when Guttmacher estimates are available.

Finally, our descriptive public health analysis of laws related to abortion access and provision in Indiana does not provide causal analysis of individual or other factors that influence Indiana's abortion rates but instead illuminates concurrent changes in abortion incidence, location, and patient characteristics over time. Our analysis is strengthened by our use of multiple large, publicly available data sets with data reported across state, regional, and national geographies.

Public Health Implications

Based on this public health description of patterns in state, regional, and national abortion rates over time, we conclude that abortion access in Indiana over the past decade was strikingly low, required increases in interstate travel to obtain care, and cooccurred with the passage of numerous abortion restrictions. With the uncertainty Indiana's contested abortion ban imposes,[43] abortion access will be even more strongly curtailed, and these findings suggest that effects may be unevenly felt, with disproportionate impact across Indiana. The change in abortion utilization seen in Indiana that coincided with legislative restrictions can serve as a potential preview of what may be expected as state-level restrictions and complete bans go into effect in additional states across the country. AJPH

ABOUT THE AUTHORS

Heidi Moseson is with Ibis Reproductive Health, Oakland, CA. Mikaela H. Smith, Hillary J. Gyuras, Abigail Foster, and Alison H. Norris are with the Ohio Policy Evaluation Network, Ohio State University, Columbus. Danielle Bessett is with the Ohio Policy Evaluation Network, University of Cincinnati, Cincinnati. Payal Chakraborty is with the Department of Population Medicine, Harvard Medical School and Harvard Pilgrim Health Care Institute, Boston, MA. Tracey A. Wilkinson is with the Indiana University School of Medicine, Indianapolis.

CORRESPONDENCE

Correspondence should be sent to Heidi Moseson, PhD, MPH, Ibis Reproductive Health, 1736 Franklin St, Suite 600, Oakland, CA 94612 (e-mail: hmoseson@ibisreproductivehealth.org). Reprints can be ordered at http://www.ajph.org by clicking the "Reprints" link.

PUBLICATION INFORMATION

Full Citation: Moseson H, Smith MH, Chakraborty P, et al. Abortion-related laws and concurrent patterns in abortion incidence in Indiana, 2010–2019. *Am J Public Health*. 2023;113(4): 429–437.

Acceptance Date: December 2, 2022.

DOI: https://doi.org/10.2105/AJPH.2022.307196

CONTRIBUTORS

H. Moseson drafted the article with support from M. H. Smith and contributions, input, and review from all authors. H. Moseson and M. H. Smith extracted and analyzed the abortion incidence data and generated the related figures. H. Moseson, M. H. Smith, D. Bessett, and A. H. Norris designed the study. P. Chakraborty conducted the geospatial analyses and generated the related figures. H. J. Gyuras and A. Foster reviewed and extracted the data on state laws and clinic closures. T. A. Wilkinson provided clinical and scientific expertise on abortion provision in Indiana and verified and interpreted the results.

ACKNOWLEDGMENTS

H. Moseson was funded by the Society of Family Planning (grant SFPRF14-MA6) and the National Cancer Institute (grant 1R21CA256759-01). M. H. Smith, P. Chakraborty, H. J. Gyuras, A. Foster, D. Bessett, and A. H. Norris were supported by a philanthropic foundation that makes grants anonymously. P. Chakraborty was also supported by the National Heart, Lung, and Blood Institute (grant T32 HL098048).

We are grateful to the staff at the Indiana State Department of Health and the United States Centers for Disease Control and Prevention for their efforts in collecting and reporting data on abortion incidence in Indiana and across the United States.

Note. The funders played no role in the design or conduct of this study or in the preparation and review of the article. The content is the responsibility of the authors and does not necessarily reflect the views of the funders.

CONFLICTS OF INTEREST

T. A. Wilkinson receives project funding from Organon, Merck, and Cooper Surgical. All authors declare no potential or actual conflicts of interest.

HUMAN PARTICIPANT PROTECTION

This study was exempt from institutional review board review under the federal regulations for human participants (45 CFR, part 46) research because this analysis involved only publicly available data sets and de-identified data.

REFERENCES

1. Guttmacher Institute. An overview of abortion laws. August 1, 2021. Available at: https://www.guttmacher.org/state-policy/explore/overview-abortion-laws. Accessed January 9, 2019.
2. US Supreme Court. *Dobbs v. Jackson Women's Health Organization.* 213 (2022). Available at: https://www.supremecourt.gov/opinions/21pdf/19-1392_6j37.pdf. Accessed January 9, 2023.
3. Guttmacher Institute. Targeted regulation of abortion providers (TRAP) laws. January 2020. Available at: https://www.guttmacher.org/evidence-you-can-use/targeted-regulation-abortion-providers-trap-laws. Accessed August 20, 2021.
4. Jerman J, Frohwirth L, Kavanaugh ML, Blades N. Barriers to abortion care and their consequences for patients traveling for services: qualitative findings from two states. *Perspect Sex Reprod Health.* 2017;49(2):95–102. https://doi.org/10.1363/psrh.12024
5. Nash E, Mohammed L, Cappello O, Naide S. State policy trends 2019: a wave of abortion bans, but some states are fighting back. 2019. Available at: https://www.guttmacher.org/article/2019/12/state-policy-trends-2019-wave-abortion-bans-some-states-are-fighting-back. Accessed September 1, 2022.
6. Nash E. State abortion policy landscape: from hostile to supportive. 2021. Available at: https://www.guttmacher.org/article/2019/08/state-abortion-policy-landscape-hostile-supportive. Accessed May 12, 2021.
7. Nash E. Louisiana has passed 89 abortion restrictions since Roe: it's about control, not health. 2020. Available at: https://www.guttmacher.org/article/2020/02/louisiana-has-passed-89-abortion-restrictions-roe-its-about-control-not-health. Accessed January 10, 2023.
8. Guttmacher Institute. State facts about abortion: Indiana. June 2020. Available at: https://www.guttmacher.org/fact-sheet/state-facts-about-abortion-indiana. Accessed February 11, 2020.
9. Indiana General Assembly. Senate Bill 1. Available at: https://iga.in.gov/legislative/2022ss1/bills/senate/1. Accessed August 30, 2022.
10. Vilda D, Wallace ME, Daniel C, Evans MG, Stoecker C, Theall KP. State abortion policies and maternal death in the United States, 2015–2018. *Am J Public Health.* 2021;111(9):1696–1704. https://doi.org/10.2105/AJPH.2021.306396
11. Foster DG. *The Turnaway Study: Ten Years, a Thousand Women, and the Consequences of Having—or Being Denied—an Abortion* . New York, NY: Simon & Schuster; 2021.
12. Ross L, Solinger R. *Reproductive Justice.* Oakland: University of California Press; 2017.
13. Gerdts C, Dobkin L, Foster DG, Schwarz EB. Side effects, physical health consequences, and mortality associated with abortion and birth after an unwanted pregnancy. *Womens Health Issues.* 2016;26(1):55–59. https://doi.org/10.1016/j.whi.2015.10.001
14. Roberts SC, Biggs MA, Chibber KS, Gould H, Rocca CH, Foster DG. Risk of violence from the man involved in the pregnancy after receiving or being denied an abortion. *BMC Med.* 2014;12(1): 144. https://doi.org/10.1186/s12916-014-0144-z
15. Foster DG, Biggs MA, Ralph L, Gerdts C, Roberts S, Glymour MM. Socioeconomic outcomes of women who receive and women who are denied wanted abortions in the United States. *Am J Public Health.* 2022;112(9):1290–1296. https://doi.org/10.2105/AJPH.2017.304247r
16. Foster DG, Biggs MA, Raifman S, Gipson J, Kimport K, Rocca CH. Comparison of health, development, maternal bonding, and poverty among children born after denial of abortion vs after pregnancies subsequent to an abortion. *JAMA Pediatr.* 2018;172(11):1053–1060. https://doi.org/10.1001/jamapediatrics.2018.1785
17. US Department of Agriculture. Rural–urban continuum codes. 2020. Available at: https://www.ers.usda.gov/data-products/rural-urban-continuum-codes. Accessed February 28, 2022.
18. US Census Bureau. American Community Survey 2015–2019 5-year data release. October 8, 2021. Available at: https://www.census.gov/newsroom/press-kits/2020/acs-5-year.html. Accessed April 12, 2022.
19. Ellertson C. Mandatory parental involvement in minors' abortions: effects of the laws in Minnesota, Missouri, and Indiana. *Am J Public Health.* 1997; 87(8):1367–1374. https://doi.org/10.2105/ajph.87.8.136720.
20. Jones RK, Witwer E, Jerman J. Abortion incidence and service availability in the United States, 2017. September 2019. Available at: https://www.guttmacher.org/report/abortion-incidence-service-availability-us-2017. Accessed May 16, 2022.
21. Centers for Disease Control and Prevention. CDCs abortion surveillance system FAQs. November 25, 2020. Available at: https://www.cdc.gov/reproductivehealth/data_stats/abortion.htm. Accessed February 12, 2021.
22. Indiana Department of Health. Terminated pregnancy reports. Available at: https://www.in.gov/health/vital-records/vital-statistics/terminated-pregnancy-reports. Accessed January 12, 2023.
23. US Census Bureau. American Community Survey 5-year data (2009–2021). December 8, 2022. Available at: https://www.census.gov/data/developers/data-sets/acs-5year.html. Accessed January 12, 2023.

24. Office of Management and Budget. Revised delineations of metropolitan statistical areas, micropolitan statistical areas, and combined statistical areas, and guidance on uses of the delineations of these areas. February 28, 2013. Available at: https://obamawhitehouse.archives.gov/sites/default/files/omb/bulletins/2013/b-13-01.pdf. Accessed February 28, 2022.
25. Smith MH, Muzyczka Z, Chakraborty P, et al. Abortion travel within the United States: an observational study of cross-state movement to obtain abortion care in 2017. *Lancet Reg Health - Am.* 2022;10:100214. https://doi.org/10.1016/j.lana.2022.100214
26. Norris AH, Chakraborty P, Lang K, et al. Abortion access in Ohio's changing legislative context, 2010–2018. *Am J Public Health.* 2020;110(8): 1228–1234. https://doi.org/10.2105/AJPH.2020.305706
27. Martins SL, Starr KA, Hellerstedt WL, Gilliam ML. Differences in family planning services by rural–urban geography: survey of Title X–supported clinics in Great Plains and Midwestern states. *Perspect Sex Reprod Health.* 2016;48(1):9–16. https://doi.org/10.1363/48e7116
28. Bennett T. Reproductive health care in the rural United States. *JAMA.* 2002;287(1):112. https://doi.org/10.1001/jama.287.1.112-JMS0102-6-1
29. Upadhyay UD, Weitz TA, Jones RK, Barar RE, Foster DG. Denial of abortion because of provider gestational age limits in the United States. *Am J Public Health.* 2014;104(9):1687–1694. https://doi.org/10.2105/AJPH.2013.301378
30. Finer LB, Frohwirth LF, Dauphinee LA, Singh S, Moore AM. Timing of steps and reasons for delays in obtaining abortions in the United States. *Contraception.* 2006;74(4):334–344. https://doi.org/10.1016/j.contraception.2006.04.010
31. Dennis A, Henshaw SK, Joyce TJ, Finer LB, Blanchard K. The impact of laws requiring parental involvement for abortion: a literature review. March 18, 2009. Available at: https://www.guttmacher.org/report/impact-laws-requiring-parental-involvement-abortion-literature-review. Accessed July 29, 2021.
32. Fuentes L, Jerman J. Distance traveled to obtain clinical abortion care in the United States and reasons for clinic choice. *J Womens Health (Larchmt).* 2019;28(12):1623–1631. https://doi.org/10.1089/jwh.2018.7496
33. Gerdts C, Fuentes L, Grossman D, et al. Impact of clinic closures on women obtaining abortion services after implementation of a restrictive law in Texas. *Am J Public Health.* 2016;106(5):857–864. https://doi.org/10.2105/AJPH.2016.303134r
34. Maddow-Zimet I, Kost K. Even before Roe was overturned, nearly one in 10 people obtaining an abortion traveled across state lines for care. July 21, 2022. Available at: https://www.guttmacher.org/article/2022/07/even-roe-was-overturned-nearly-one-10-people-obtaining-abortion-traveled-across. Accessed August 19, 2022.
35. Joffe C, Parker WJ. Race, reproductive politics and reproductive health care in the contemporary United States. *Contraception.* 2012;86(1):1–3. https://doi.org/10.1016/j.contraception.2012.03.009
36. Dehlendorf C, Weitz T. Access to abortion services: a neglected health disparity. *J Health Care Poor Underserved.* 2011;22(2):415–421. https://doi.org/10.1353/hpu.2011.0064
37. Thompson TM, Young YY, Bass TM, et al. Racism runs through it: examining the sexual and reproductive health experience of Black women in the South. *Health Aff (Millwood).* 2022;41(2):195–202. https://doi.org/10.1377/hlthaff.2021.01422
38. Troutman M, Rafique S, Plowden TC. Are higher unintended pregnancy rates among minorities a result of disparate access to contraception? *Contracept Reprod Med.* 2020;5:16. https://doi.org/10.1186/s40834-020-00118-5
39. Roberts DE. *Killing the Black Body: Race, Reproduction, and the Meaning of Liberty.* New York: Vintage; 1997.
40. Harris LH, Wolfe T. Stratified reproduction, family planning care and the double edge of history. *Curr Opin Obstet Gynecol.* 2014;26(6):539–544. https://doi.org/10.1097/GCO.0000000000000121
41. Solazzo AL. Different and not equal: the uneven association of race, poverty, and abortion laws on abortion timing. *Soc Probl.* 2019;66(4):519–547. https://doi.org/10.1093/socpro/spy015
42. Moseson H, Seymour JW, Zuniga C, et al. "It just seemed like a perfect storm": a multi-methods feasibility study on the use of Facebook, Google Ads, and Reddit to collect data on abortion-seeking experiences from people who considered but did not obtain abortion care in the United States. *PLoS One.* 2022;17(3):e0264748. https://doi.org/10.1371/journal.pone.0264748
43. Stracqualursi V. Judge blocks Indiana's near-total abortion ban. *CNN.* September 22, 2022. Available at: https://www.cnn.com/2022/09/22/politics/indiana-abortion-ban-blocked/index.html. Accessed September 23, 2022.

Impact of School Shootings on Adolescent School Safety, 2009–2019

James C. Hodges, MSW, LCSW, Danielle T. Walker, MSN, PMHNP-BC, Christopher F. Baum, PhD, and Summer Sherburne Hawkins, PhD, MS

Objectives. To examine the impact of school shootings on indicators of adolescent school safety in the United States.

Methods. We linked 2009–2019 Youth Risk Behavior Survey data on 211 236 adolescents aged 14 to 18 years from 24 school districts with data on high school shootings from the Center for Homeland Defense and Security. We conducted 2-way fixed-effects logistic regression models to assess the impact of shootings on self-report of 3 indicators of school safety: avoiding school because of feeling unsafe, carrying a weapon at school, and being threatened or injured with a weapon at school.

Results. High school shootings were associated with adolescents having 20% greater odds of avoiding school because of feeling unsafe (adjusted odd ratio [AOR] = 1.20; 95% confidence interval [CI] = 1.11, 1.29) than those who had not. Findings were slightly attenuated in sensitivity analyses that tested exposure to shootings at any school in the district or state. High school shootings were associated with a statistically nonsignificant ($P = .08$) elevated risk of carrying a weapon at school (AOR = 1.11; 95% CI = 0.99, 1.25).

Conclusions. The negative ramifications of school shootings extend far beyond the event itself to adolescents' concerns about school safety. (*Am J Public Health*. 2023;113(4):438–441. https://doi.org/10.2105/AJPH.2022.307206)

AJPH April 2023, Vol 113, No. 4

In 2020, firearm-related deaths were the leading cause of mortality for children and adolescents, with more than 3500 youths dying by gun violence.[1,2] School shootings have also increased, peaking in 2018 and 2019, with 75 shootings occurring annually.[3] Over recent years, almost one third of states have weakened their gun laws,[4] which has implications for adolescent health.

Ghiani et al. found that states that adopted stricter gun laws decreased the likelihood of adolescents avoiding school because of safety concerns or of carrying or being threatened by weapons at school.[5] However, whether exposure to school shootings is associated with these behaviors remains unknown. Using representative samples across 24 school districts, we examined the impact of school shootings on 3 indicators of adolescent school safety: avoiding school because of feeling unsafe, carrying a weapon at school, and being threatened by a weapon at school.

METHODS

We used repeated cross-sectional data from the 2009–2019 Youth Risk Behavior Survey (YRBS) biennial school district surveys, which collect self-reported health-related behaviors on 9th through 12th graders in public and private schools.[6] Among the 31 districts that participated across study years with at least 2 years of data collection, we excluded 7 because the Centers for Disease Control and Prevention did not have permission to release the data. Our analytic sample included 211 236 adolescents aged 14 to 18 years from 24 districts that collected information on 3 outcomes: (1) number of days not attending school because of feeling unsafe at school or on the way to or from school during the past month, (2) number of days carrying a weapon on school property during the past month, and (3) number of times threatened or injured with a weapon on school property during the past year. Each outcome was dichotomized (0 vs ≥ 1), and analytic samples were based on available responses for each outcome measure.

We obtained school shootings data from the Center for Homeland Defense and Security from April 2007 to March 2019, which we defined as shootings resulting in an injury or death that occurred at any high school in the district.[7] We linked the shootings to each adolescent based on whether the event occurred between April 1 of the previous survey year to March 31 of the current survey year, as the YRBS is administered biennially in the spring.[6] We dichotomized school shootings (0 vs ≥ 1) for each survey period.

We first examined the associations between demographic characteristics (age, gender, race/ethnicity) and each outcome using adjusted logistic regression models with year and district fixed effects. Next, we conducted 2-way fixed-effects logistic regression models to assess the impact of school shootings on each indicator of school safety, controlling for demographics with year and district fixed effects. We tested interactions between school shootings and age, gender, and race/ethnicity using the Wald test. Only 1 interaction was jointly significant ($P < .05$), but none of the stratum-specific estimates were significant (results not shown).

We conducted 2 sensitivity analyses: (1) shootings that occurred at any elementary, middle, or high school in the district; (2) shootings that occurred at any school in the state. We also conducted 2 robustness checks with the main model (results not shown). We first included county-level indicators of percentage Black, percentage Hispanic, and ratio of 90th to 10th percentile of income,[8] but none of the factors had any effect. Second, we included an indicator of any school shooting in the prior 2 to 4 years (i.e., in the prior wave), but it did not alter the effect size or the significance of exposure to recent shootings.

We conducted analyses using Stata statistical software version 17.0 (StataCorp LP, College Station, TX), with robust standard errors and survey weights to account for the cluster sampling design.[6]

RESULTS

Over the study period, 17 of 24 school districts experienced at least 1 shooting, with a total of 56 shootings across districts (Table A, available as a supplement to the online version of this article at http://www.ajph.org). Overall, 9.2% of adolescents reported avoiding school because of feeling unsafe, 3.5% reported carrying a weapon at school, and 7.3% reported being threatened with a weapon at school. Age was positively associated with each outcome, and males were less likely to avoid school because of feeling unsafe than females but more likely to have weapon exposure (Table B, available as a supplement to the online version of this article at http://www.ajph.org). Black and Hispanic adolescents were more likely to report all outcomes than White adolescents.

We found that being exposed to high school shootings was associated with adolescents having 20% greater odds of avoiding school because of feeling unsafe (adjusted odds ratio [AOR] = 1.20; 95% confidence interval [CI] = 1.11, 1.29) than those who had not (Table 1). Findings were consistent, but slightly attenuated, in sensitivity analyses that tested exposure to shootings at any school in the district or state.

We found some evidence that high school shootings were associated with an elevated risk of carrying a weapon at school (AOR = 1.11; 95% CI = 0.99, 1.25), but at a P level of .08 (Table 1). There were no effects of shootings on being threatened with a weapon at school. The alternative specifications were not significant for either outcome.

DISCUSSION

Adolescents exposed to school shootings in their district or state were more likely to avoid at least 1 day of school during the past month because of feeling unsafe compared with adolescents who were not. We found some evidence, albeit marginally significant, that adolescents were more likely to carry weapons at school in response to shootings. Although school safety outcomes varied by age, gender, and race/ethnicity, the effects of shootings did not vary across these characteristics. These results extend previous work[5] by demonstrating that simply being exposed to school shootings increases adolescents' school avoidance because of feeling unsafe and, possibly, increases weapon carrying at school.

Using large, representative samples of adolescents linked with government data, our work highlights that the negative ramifications of school shootings extend far beyond the event itself.[9] These effects are evident for exposure to shootings that occur not only in high schools within the district that adolescents attend school, but in any type of school in their district or state. Because of ever-expanding news coverage and social media, exposure to such events beyond school districts will likely increase.

Despite these strengths, limitations remain. Outcomes were self-reported and subject to reporting bias. Because our analysis included only 24 school districts, the findings may not be

TABLE 1— Impact of School Shootings on Adolescent School Safety and Weapon Exposure: United States, Youth Risk Behavior Survey, 2009–2019

	Avoiding School Because of Feeling Unsafe, AOR[a] (95% CI)	Carrying Weapon at School, AOR[a] (95% CI)	Being Threatened by Weapon at School, AOR[a] (95% CI)
School shooting at any high school in the district	1.20 (1.11, 1.29)	1.11 (0.99, 1.25)	1.03 (0.95, 1.12)
School shooting at any school in the district[b]	1.15 (1.07, 1.23)	1.08 (0.98, 1.21)	1.04 (0.97, 1.13)
Any school shooting in the state[b]	1.18 (1.08, 1.29)	1.00 (0.89, 1.13)	0.96 (0.88, 1.04)

Note. AOR = adjusted odds ratio; CI = confidence interval. For more details, see Table A (available as a supplement to the online version of this article at http://www.ajph.org).

[a]Model adjusted for age, gender, race/ethnicity, year, and district fixed effects.
[b]Includes elementary, middle, and high schools.

generalizable to all high school students. Although the YRBS collects limited demographic information, we found that county-level indicators of race/ethnicity and income were not associated with any outcomes other than individual-level factors. The YRBS also does not release school identifiers, so it was not possible to isolate the effects of attending the actual school where a shooting occurred, or whether adolescents moved into the district after the shooting took place. We could not control for community-based violence, which may affect school safety. Because the YRBS is cross-sectional, we were also not able to follow adolescents over time. The YRBS was administered in school, and students who avoided school because of feeling unsafe may be underrepresented in the data set if they were absent on the day of the survey. This suggests that our findings may underestimate the true association between experiencing a shooting firsthand and adolescent concerns about school safety.

PUBLIC HEALTH IMPLICATIONS

School shootings are disturbingly common, occurring in more than 70% of the included districts. Our results highlight that, with firearm violence on the rise,[1] health care providers need to screen for the educational and psychosocial sequelae of these events. Furthermore, screening should occur for adolescents who attend neighboring schools or adjacent districts with a shooting, in addition to those in the immediate vicinity, as the adverse effects appear to extend well beyond the schools where the shooting occurs. For these districts, a universal, trauma-informed approach to providing psychosocial support to adolescents appears warranted. Our findings also underscore the need for continued advocacy to implement policies that reduce school shootings and gun-related violence, as they have previously been found to reduce adverse outcomes.[5] Minimizing the number of adolescents affected by these horrific events remains a public health imperative. AJPH

ABOUT THE AUTHORS

James C. Hodges and Summer Sherburne Hawkins are with the School of Social Work, Danielle T. Walker is with the William F. Connell School of Nursing, and Christopher F. Baum is with the Department of Economics and School of Social Work, Boston College, Chestnut Hill, MA. Christopher F. Baum is also with the Department of Macroeconomics, German Institute for Economic Research (DIW Berlin), Berlin, Germany.

CORRESPONDENCE

Correspondence should be sent to Summer Sherburne Hawkins, PhD, MS, Boston College, School of Social Work, McGuinn Hall, 140 Commonwealth Ave, Chestnut Hill, MA 02467 (e-mail: summer.hawkins@bc.edu). Reprints can be ordered at http://www.ajph.org by clicking the "Reprints" link.

PUBLICATION INFORMATION

Full Citation: Hodges JC, Walker DT, Baum CF, Hawkins SS. Impact of school shootings on adolescent school safety, 2009–2019. *Am J Public Health*. 2023;113(4):438–441.

Acceptance Date: December 10, 2022

DOI: https://doi.org/10.2105/AJPH.2022.307206

CONTRIBUTORS

J. C. Hodges and D. T. Walker are joint first authors and contributed equally to this article. S. S. Hawkins conceptualized and designed the study. J. C. Hodges and C. F. Baum procured the data and carried out the analyses. J. C. Hodges and D. T. Walker contributed to the initial draft of the article. All the authors reviewed and edited the article.

CONFLICTS OF INTEREST

The authors have no conflicts of interest to declare.

HUMAN PARTICIPANT PROTECTION

The Boston College institutional review board reviewed this study and considered it exempt.

REFERENCES

1. Goldstick JE, Cunningham RM, Carter PM. Current causes of death in children and adolescents in the United States. *N Engl J Med*. 2022;386(20):1955–1956. https://doi.org/10.1056/NEJMc2201761
2. Everytown Research & Policy. The impact of gun violence on children and teens. Updated December 28, 2021. Available at: https://everytownresearch.

org/report/the-impact-of-gun-violence-on-children-and-teens. Accessed June 17, 2022.

3. National Center for Education Statistics. Violent deaths at school and away from school and school shootings. US Dept of Education, Institute of Education Sciences. Updated May 2022. Available at: https://nces.ed.gov/programs/coe/indicator/a01. Accessed June 17, 2022.
4. State Firearm Laws Project. State firearm law database. Available at: http://statefirearmlaws.org. Accessed June 27, 2022.
5. Ghiani M, Hawkins SS, Baum CF. Gun laws and school safety. *J Epidemiol Community Health.* 2019; 73(6):509–515. https://doi.org/10.1136/jech-2018-211246
6. Underwood JM, Brener N, Thornton J, et al. Overview and methods for the Youth Risk Behavior Surveillance System—United States, 2019. *MMWR Suppl.* 2020;69(1):1–10. https://doi.org/10.15585/mmwr.su6901a1
7. Center for Homeland Defense and Security. K-12 school shooting database. Available at: https://www.chds.us/ssdb. Accessed June 24, 2022.
8. US Census Bureau. American Community Survey Data. Updated November 23, 2021. Available at: https://www.census.gov/programs-surveys/acs/data.html. Accessed June 6, 2022.
9. Lowe SR, Galea S. The mental health consequences of mass shootings. *Trauma Violence Abuse.* 2017;18(1):62–82. https://doi.org/10.1177/1524838015591572

Housing Instability and Evictions Linked to Elevated Intimate Partner and Workplace Violence Among Women Sex Workers in Vancouver, Canada: Findings of a Prospective, Community-Based Cohort, 2010–2019

Shira M. Goldenberg, PhD, MSc, Natalie Buglioni, MPH, Andrea Krüsi, PhD, MPH, Elizabeth Frost, MSW, Sarah Moreheart, MPH, Melissa Braschel, MSc, and Kate Shannon, PhD, MPH

AJPH April 2023, Vol 113, No. 4

Objectives. To model the relationship of unstable housing and evictions with physical and sexual violence perpetrated against women sex workers in intimate and workplace settings.

Methods. We used bivariate and multivariable logistic regression with generalized estimating equations to model the association of unstable housing exposure and evictions with intimate partner violence (IPV) and workplace violence among a community-based longitudinal cohort of cisgender and transgender women sex workers in Vancouver, Canada, from 2010 through 2019.

Results. Of 946 women, 85.9% experienced unstable housing, 11.1% eviction, 26.2% IPV, and 31.8% workplace violence. In multivariable generalized estimating equation models, recent exposure to unstable housing (adjusted odds ratio [AOR] = 2.04; 95% confidence interval [CI] = 1.45, 2.87) and evictions (AOR = 2.45; 95% CI = 0.99, 6.07) were associated with IPV, and exposure to unstable housing was associated with workplace violence (AOR = 1.46; 95% CI = 1.06, 2.00).

Conclusions. Women sex workers face a high burden of unstable housing and evictions, which are linked to increased odds of intimate partner and workplace violence. Increased access to safe, women-centered, and nondiscriminatory housing is urgently needed. (*Am J Public Health*. 2023;113(4):442–452. https://doi.org/10.2105/AJPH.2022.307207)

Housing is a critical social determinant of health and well-being and has been described as a key pathway through which health inequities emerge and are sustained over time.[1] In recent years, Vancouver, Canada, like many other places in North America, has experienced an intensifying housing crisis. Community concerns regarding affordable and appropriate housing have continued to intensify, as low-income family housing, single-room occupancy hotels, and social housing continue to be upscaled or replaced by new housing and retail units.

Women sex workers often face intense marginalization stemming from criminalization, stigma and discrimination, and limited labor protections. These are all structural factors that have been strongly associated with an elevated burden of violence among sex workers, including both occupational and intimate partner violence (IPV).[2,3] The estimated prevalence of workplace violence (i.e., physical or sexual violence perpetuated against sex workers) in the past 6 months is 50% to 70% for physical violence and 80% for sexual violence.[4] In regard to IPV, an estimated 60% of women sex workers have experienced physical violence and 40% have experienced sexual violence over their lifetimes.[4]

In comparison with the general population, sex workers face disproportionate risks related to housing instability and evictions because of structural factors, including pervasive criminalization and stigma.[5,6] Despite growing concerns regarding the negative health and social consequences of unaffordable housing and, in particular, evictions amid the COVID-19 pandemic,[7,8] epidemiologic data are lacking on the role of housing instability and evictions as structural determinants of violence across both intimate partner and occupational contexts among sex workers. This information is needed to inform housing-centered interventions for marginalized women. Previous literature suggests that women experiencing IPV may be more likely to face housing precarity.[9–13] Research from Baltimore, Maryland,[11] and Vancouver[12] documents associations of homelessness with younger age, drug use, sexual IPV, client volume, and working in public or outdoor workplaces.

Research on housing and marginalized women's health has focused mainly on homelessness, which is the most visible and commonly studied form of housing precarity and, more narrowly, refers to experiences of being unhoused or unsheltered. However, less attention has been paid to the needs of marginalized women affected by other forms of housing precarity, such as evictions and housing instability. We define "housing instability" as requiring temporary or marginal overnight sleeping arrangements—such as in a shelter, a hotel, supportive housing, a car, or a recovery house; on the street; with family or friends; or couch surfing—that could lead to loss of housing and eventual homelessness. We operationalize "eviction" as changing one's place of living or sleeping owing to being evicted or forced to move by one's landlord or housing operator. Research has found that some types of sleeping arrangements (e.g., couch surfing) among those experiencing homelessness are more common for youths and are associated with deleterious mental and physical health outcomes.[14,15]

Previous qualitative literature has described housing as a critical determinant shaping marginalized women's health and safety. Women who use drugs and experience poverty report frequent exposure to rental discrimination, gender-based violence, exploitation, and lack of security and privacy in traditional co-ed low-income housing settings (e.g., single-room occupancy hotels). These inequities may be heightened for transgender women.[16,17] Furthermore, the criminalization of aspects of sex work can result in rental discrimination, such as proprietors being less likely to rent to and more likely to evict sex workers.[6] Additionally, in the absence of a safe place to take dates, sexual transactions may be relegated to unsafe or isolated settings where sex workers have few protections from occupational violence.[6,18] However, few epidemiological studies have analyzed housing instability or evictions in relation to health and safety outcomes, particularly experiences of violence, among women sex workers.[19,20] Such research remains critically needed given previous work that has highlighted strong links between IPV and housing precarity among women in the general population and that shows that women experiencing violence are often forced to rely on provisional, overcrowded, or unaffordable housing.[21]

Building on previous research indicating a high burden of homelessness[12] and of violence[22,23] in intimate partner and occupational settings among women sex workers, we assessed the independent association of exposure to unstable housing and evictions with IPV and occupational violence among women sex workers in Vancouver, Canada, over a 9-year study period (2010–2019).

METHODS

We collected data from An Evaluation of Sex Workers Health Access (AESHA), an open longitudinal community-based cohort of sex workers in Vancouver, Canada. AESHA is overseen by a community advisory board of 15 or more community agencies. Eligibility criteria were self-identifying as a woman (cisgender and transgender inclusive), being aged 14 years or older, having exchanged sex for money in the past 30 days in Metro Vancouver, and being able to provide informed consent. We recruited participants through time–space sampling, as described previously,[24] across various workplaces (e.g., streets, indoor venues) and online. After providing written informed consent, participants completed baseline and biannual study visits composed of an interviewer-administered questionnaire and serological testing. Visits took place at participants' location of choice (i.e., study office or women's homes or workplaces) and were conducted by experienced (current or former sex workers) and community-based interviewers and clinical staff. We used Biolytical INSTI (Biolytical Laboratories, Inc., Richmond, BC) rapid tests for HIV screening, with confirmation of reactive tests by blood draw for Western blot. We collected urine samples to test for gonorrhea and chlamydia, and drew blood to test for syphilis, HSV-2 (herpes simplex virus 2) antibody, and HCV (hepatitis C).

Project nurses provided pre- and posttest counseling as well as treatment of symptomatic sexually transmitted infections onsite and offered referrals for HIV care to participants living with HIV. Serology and Papanicolaou testing were available to community members regardless of study participation. Participants received an honorarium of 40.00 CAD (Canadian dollars) per study visit.

Measures

We assessed demographics and other lifetime exposures using baseline data only; for other study variables (e.g., housing, violence, substance use), we used time-updated data, examining events with recall periods in the past 6 months at baseline and each biannual study visit. Except for age, income, and place of solicitation, all study variables were binary.

Housing exposure variables. We defined "unstable housing" with participants' response to the question "In which of the following types of places have you slept overnight in the last six months?" We coded having temporary or marginal housing experiences in the past 6 months (e.g., street, shelter, hostel, hotel, supportive housing, car, family or friends, couch surfing, recovery house) as "yes." We coded permanent housing (e.g., living in apartment or house on own or with others) as "no." We evaluated evictions with participants' response to the question "Have you changed the main place where you live or sleep overnight in the last 6 months? If yes, why?" We coded women who changed their place of living or sleeping because of being evicted or forced to move in the past 6 months as "yes." Those who did not change their place of living or sleeping or who did so for reasons other than evictions made up the comparison group. We measured unstable housing across the duration of the study (January 2010–February 2019), and we collected data on evictions from September 2014 through February 2019.

Violence outcomes. As with previous research,[22] we defined IPV as moderate to severe physical or sexual violence perpetrated by any male intimate partners in the past 6 months, as measured on the World Health Organization Intimate Partner Violence Scale.[25] We evaluated IPV based on participants' response to the question "Have you ever experienced any of the following by your intimate male partners (boyfriends, spouse) in the past six months?" Types of IPV were "moderate physical IPV" (e.g., being slapped, thrown at, pushed, or shoved); "severe physical IPV" (e.g., being hit, kicked, dragged, beaten, choked, or burned); and "sexual IPV" (e.g., being forced to have sex against one's will). We considered women who responded yes to any of the measures of violence to have experienced IPV.

Workplace violence consisted of physical or sexual violence perpetrated by aggressors posing as clients. We evaluated workplace violence based on participants' response to the question "Have you experienced any of the following bad dates or experienced violence by clients in the past six months?" We considered women who reported any experiences of physical or sexual violence perpetrated by aggressors posing as clients (e.g., abduction or kidnap, sexual or physical assault or rape, strangulation, or being locked or trapped in a car or room) to have experienced workplace violence.

Potential confounders. Time-fixed (i.e., lifetime) covariates assessed only at baseline were age (in years), educational attainment (whether graduated from high school), Indigenous ancestry (First Nations, Metis, or Inuit ancestry), whether immigrant to Canada (i.e., born outside Canada), sexual orientation (gay, lesbian, bisexual, two spirit, asexual, or queer vs straight), gender identity (transgender woman, transexual woman, or other transfeminine identity vs cisgender woman), whether ever diagnosed with a mental health condition (yes vs no), and whether experienced childhood trauma (i.e., physical or sexual assault before 18 years old).

Time-updated confounders included noninjection (excluding alcohol and cannabis) and injection drug use, inconsistent condom use with clients, client condom refusal, being forced to have sex against will with clients, having experienced sexual assault (by anyone other than intimate partners or clients), and having experienced violence from community members (verbal harassment or physical violence by community residents or business owners). Time-updated structural factors were average monthly income from all sources (in CAD), having access to health care services when needed, always or usually having privacy where currently living, ever feeling in danger where currently sleeping, primary place of solicitation, having experienced police harassment while working (excluding arrest), and incarceration (i.e., in detention, prison, or jail overnight or longer).

We defined primary place of solicitation as 1 of 3 mutually exclusive categories: street or public space, indoor establishment (e.g., crack or drug house; bar, nightclub, or strip club; massage or beauty parlor; microbrothel; single-room occupancy hotel or supportive housing), and independent (e.g., escort agency, newspaper ads, online or

AJPH April 2023, Vol 113, No. 4

telephone or texting, arranged by third party). Police harassment consisted of a range of harmful policing practices (e.g., being threatened with arrest, detainment, or fine; verbal harassment; physical assault; confiscation of harm-reduction materials; coercion into providing sexual favors).

Statistical Analyses

We restricted analyses to observations for which participants reported active engagement in sex work in the past 6 months at each study visit (2010–2019). We restricted models examining IPV to observations for which participants had at least 1 intimate male partner in the past 6 months. We further restricted analyses of evictions to participants interviewed after these questions were added (September 2014–February 2019).

We examined descriptive statistics at baseline, stratified by outcomes in the past 6 months at baseline (i.e., unstable housing and evictions). We used the Pearson χ^2 test (or the Fisher exact test for small cell counts) for categorical variables and the Wilcoxon rank–sum test for continuous variables to test for significant differences between participants who had and those who had not experienced the outcome of interest. We conducted all bivariate and multivariable analyses using logistic regression with generalized estimating equations (GEE) and an exchangeable correlation matrix. We first used bivariate analyses to examine associations between hypothesized exposures and outcomes. To examine independent effects of housing exposures (i.e., unstable housing and evictions) on violence outcomes (i.e., IPV and workplace violence), we developed 4 separate multivariable GEE logistic regression confounder models using the procedure described by Maldonado and Greenland.[26]

We included key confounders that we identified in bivariate analyses and hypothesized to impact gender-based violence outcomes as potential confounders in full models. To determine the most parsimonious models, we removed potential confounders in a stepwise manner. We removed all potential confounding variables that altered the association of interest by less than 5% from models. We performed all analyses using SAS version 9.4 (SAS, Cary, NC). All *P* values were 2 sided.

RESULTS

Analyses of unstable housing included 4765 observations among 946 participants interviewed from January 2010 through February 2019. Over the study period, the majority (85.9%) of participants experienced unstable housing (3796 events), and 45.7% reported feeling in danger where they slept. Participants reported a high burden of violence over the 9-year study, with 26.2% experiencing IPV (451 events) and 31.8% experiencing workplace violence (552 events) in the past 6 months at any study visit. Analyses of evictions included 1891 observations among 550 participants interviewed from September 2014 through February 2019. Among participants who answered questions about evictions from September 2014 through February 2019, 11.1% experienced eviction (74 events) at least once over a 4.5-year period.

At baseline, the median income was $3000 CAD per month (interquartile range [IQR] = $1790–$5620), and 55.6% had graduated from high school (Table 1); 31.9% reported minority sexual orientation, and 38.1% were of Indigenous ancestry. Two thirds (66.2%) had used noninjection drugs and 40.7% had used injection drugs in the past 6 months. Almost half (48.7%) of participants reported soliciting on the street or in public, whereas 30.2% solicited services in indoor establishments, and 20.4% solicited services independently at baseline.

At baseline, younger participants were more likely to have experienced unstable housing (34 years; IQR = 27–42 vs 37 years; IQR = 31–43) and evictions (35 years; IQR = 30–42 vs 40 years; IQR = 31–47) than were older participants (Tables 1 and 2). We also observed higher proportions of unstable housing and evictions among those identifying as gender and sexual minorities. Indigenous participants were more likely to have experienced unstable housing (46.9% vs 13.3%) and evictions (63.0% vs 42.8%) than were non-Indigenous women.

Women who used noninjection (82.5% vs 20.5%) and injection (52.1% vs 8.8%) drugs were significantly more likely to experience unstable housing, which followed a similar pattern for evictions (85.2% vs 58.5% and 66.7% vs 44.7%, respectively). Women diagnosed with mental illness were more likely to experience unstable housing (58.3% vs 24.1%) and evictions (74.1% vs 56.4%). A higher proportion of women who solicited on the street or in public spaces experienced unstable housing (61.7% vs 12.5%) and evictions (70.4% vs 36.9%), a pattern that was reversed for women who solicited in indoor establishments (14.6% vs 73.9% for unstable housing and 3.7% vs 26.4% for evictions).

In separate multivariable GEE confounder models (Table 3) adjusted for confounders (e.g., childhood trauma, Indigenous ancestry, drug use), exposure to recent unstable housing was significantly correlated with elevated odds of both recent IPV (adjusted odds

TABLE 1— Baseline Characteristics of Women Sex Workers Who Experienced Unstable Housing in the Past 6 Months Compared With Those Who Did Not: Vancouver, Canada, 2010–2019

Characteristic	Total (n = 946), No. (%) or Median (IQR)	Experienced Unstable Housing (n = 697), No. (%) or Median (IQR)	Did Not Experience Unstable Housing (n = 249), No. (%) or Median (IQR)	P
Lifetime variables				
Age, y	35 (28–42)	34 (27–42)	37 (31–43)	< .001
Minority sexual orientation				< .001
Yes	302 (31.9)	260 (37.3)	42 (16.9)	
No	642 (67.9)	436 (62.6)	206 (82.7)	
Transgender woman				.026
Yes	58 (6.1)	50 (7.2)	8 (3.2)	
No	886 (93.7)	646 (92.7)	240 (96.4)	
Indigenous				< .001
Yes	360 (38.1)	327 (46.9)	33 (13.3)	
No	585 (61.8)	370 (53.1)	215 (86.4)	
Mental health diagnosis ever				< .001
Yes	466 (49.3)	406 (58.3)	60 (24.1)	
No	480 (50.7)	291 (41.8)	189 (75.9)	
Experienced childhood trauma				< .001
Yes	635 (67.1)	552 (79.2)	83 (33.3)	
No	38 (4.0)	30 (4.3)	8 (3.2)	
Graduated from high school				< .001
Yes	526 (55.6)	333 (47.8)	193 (77.5)	
No	420 (44.4)	364 (52.2)	56 (22.5)	
Immigrated or migrated to Canada				< .001
Yes	277 (29.3)	101 (14.5)	176 (70.7)	
No	668 (70.6)	596 (85.5)	72 (28.9)	
Recent variables (occurrences in past 6 mo)				
Experienced IPV				< .001
Yes	135 (14.3)	129 (18.5)	6 (2.4)	
No	777 (3.6)	535 (76.8)	242 (97.2)	
Experienced workplace violence				< .001
Yes	168 (17.8)	153 (22.0)	15 (6.0)	
No	764 (80.8)	530 (76.0)	234 (94.0)	
Noninjection drug use				< .001
Yes	627 (66.3)	576 (82.6)	51 (20.5)	
No	317 (33.5)	119 (17.1)	198 (79.5)	
Injection drug use				< .001
Yes	384 (40.7)	362 (52.1)	22 (8.8)	
No	561 (59.3)	334 (47.9)	227 (91.2)	
Inconsistent condom use				< .001
Yes	167 (17.7)	153 (22.0)	14 (5.6)	
No	764 (80.8)	532 (76.3)	232 (93.2)	
Client condom refusal				< .001
Yes	196 (20.7)	171 (24.5)	25 (10.0)	
No	719 (76.0)	499 (71.6)	220 (88.3)	

Continued

TABLE 1— Continued

Characteristic	Total (n = 946), No. (%) or Median (IQR)	Experienced Unstable Housing (n = 697), No. (%) or Median (IQR)	Did Not Experience Unstable Housing (n = 249), No. (%) or Median (IQR)	P
Forced into sex against will				<.001
Yes	67 (7.1)	61 (8.8)	6 (2.4)	
No	864 (91.3)	622 (89.2)	242 (97.2)	
Experienced sexual assault				.003
Yes	23 (2.4)	23 (3.3)	0 (0.0)	
No	902 (95.4)	653 (93.7)	249 (100.0)	
Experienced violence from community				<.001
Yes	153 (16.2)	144 (20.7)	9 (3.6)	
No	791 (83.6)	551 (79.1)	240 (96.4)	
Has access to health services				.14
Yes	804 (85.0)	600 (86.1)	204 (81.9)	
No	137 (14.5)	94 (13.5)	43 (17.3)	
Has privacy where they live				<.001
Yes	651 (68.8)	448 (64.3)	203 (81.5)	
No	286 (30.2)	242 (34.7)	44 (17.7)	
Primary place of solicitation				<.001
Street or public space	461 (48.7)	430 (61.7)	31 (12.5)	
Indoor establishment	286 (30.2)	102 (14.6)	184 (73.9)	
Independent	193 (20.4)	159 (22.8)	34 (13.7)	
Experienced police harassment				<.001
Yes	295 (31.2)	259 (37.2)	36 (14.5)	
No	649 (68.6)	436 (62.6)	213 (85.5)	
Monthly income, CAD	3000 (1790–5620)	3000 (1730–5910)	3085 (2000–4800)	.7

Note. CAD = Canadian dollars; IPV = intimate partner violence; IQR = interquartile range.

ratio [AOR] = 2.04; 95% CI = 1.45, 2.87) and workplace violence (AOR = 1.46; 95% CI = 1.06, 2.00) over the 9-year period (2014–2019). Additionally, exposure to recent eviction was associated with increased odds of recent IPV (AOR = 2.45; 95% CI = 0.99, 6.07) over a 4.5-year period (2014–2019) after adjustment for key confounders (e.g., age, childhood trauma abuse, income). Evictions were not significantly associated with workplace violence in GEE analyses.

DISCUSSION

We have documented a high burden of unstable housing and evictions in a diverse cohort of women sex workers in Metro Vancouver, British Columbia, Canada. Housing instability was associated with increased odds of intimate partner and workplace violence, and evictions were further associated with increased odds of IPV. More than three quarters of sex workers faced housing insecurity, almost half reported feeling in danger where they slept, and 1 in 10 experienced eviction.

We also documented a high prevalence of gender-based violence, with more than one quarter of women reporting recent IPV and almost one third reporting recent workplace violence. These human rights violations highlight housing precarity as an important form of institutionalized discrimination faced by sex workers and highlight the need for urgent policy reforms—including decriminalization of sex work—to support access to safe, stable, and nondiscriminatory housing options for women sex workers. This is particularly important for reducing inequities in housing and health faced by marginalized subgroups that our analysis showed experienced a higher burden of unstable housing and evictions. These subgroups include sexual and gender minorities, youths, Indigenous women, women who use drugs, and women with mental health diagnoses.

TABLE 2— Baseline Characteristics of Women Sex Workers Who Experienced Eviction in the Past 6 Months Compared With Those Who Did Not: Vancouver, Canada, 2014–2019

Characteristic	Total (n = 550), No. (%) or Median (IQR)	Evicted (n = 27), No. (%) or Median (IQR)	Not Evicted (n = 523), No. (%) or Median (IQR)	P
Lifetime variables				
Age, y	39 (31–46)	35 (30–42)	40 (31–47)	.028
Minority sexual orientation				.13
Yes	210 (38.2)	14 (51.9)	196 (37.5)	
No	340 (61.8)	13 (48.2)	327 (62.5)	
Transgender woman				.5
Yes	47 (8.6)	3 (11.1)	44 (8.4)	
No	503 (91.5)	24 (88.9)	479 (91.6)	
Indigenous				.041
Yes	241 (43.8)	17 (63.0)	224 (42.8)	
No	308 (56.0)	10 (37.0)	298 (57.0)	
Mental health diagnosis ever				.07
Yes	315 (57.3)	20 (74.1)	295 (56.4)	
No	235 (42.7)	7 (25.9)	228 (43.6)	
Experienced childhood trauma				.003
Yes	392 (71.3)	27 (100)	365 (69.8)	
No	125 (22.7)	0 (0)	125 (23.9)	
Graduated from high school				.9
Yes	294 (53.5)	15 (55.6)	279 (53.4)	
No	256 (46.6)	12 (44.4)	244 (46.7)	
Immigrated or migrated to Canada				.08
Yes	139 (25.3)	3 (11.1)	136 (26.0)	
No	410 (74.6)	24 (88.9)	386 (73.8)	
Recent variables (occurrences in past 6 mo)				
Experienced IPV				.017
Yes	46 (8.4)	6 (22.2)	40 (7.7)	
No	476 (86.6)	19 (70.4)	457 (87.4)	
Experienced workplace violence				.5
Yes	41 (7.5)	3 (11.1)	38 (7.3)	
No	498 (90.6)	24 (88.9)	474 (90.6)	
Noninjection drug use				.006
Yes	329 (59.8)	23 (85.2)	306 (58.5)	
No	220 (40.0)	4 (14.8)	216 (41.3)	
Injection drug use				.026
Yes	252 (45.8)	18 (66.7)	234 (44.7)	
No	297 (54.0)	9 (33.3)	288 (55.1)	
Inconsistent condom use				.3
Yes	95 (17.3)	7 (25.9)	88 (16.8)	
No	444 (80.7)	20 (74.1)	424 (81.1)	
Client condom refusal				.3
Yes	81 (14.7)	6 (22.2)	75 (14.3)	
No	448 (81.5)	20 (74.1)	428 (81.8)	

Continued

TABLE 2— Continued

Characteristic	Total (n = 550), No. (%) or Median (IQR)	Evicted (n = 27), No. (%) or Median (IQR)	Not Evicted (n = 523), No. (%) or Median (IQR)	P
Forced into sex against will				.1
Yes	24 (4.4)	3 (11.1)	21 (4.0)	
No	515 (93.6)	22 (81.5)	493 (94.3)	
Experienced sexual assault				.12
Yes	12 (2.2)	2 (7.4)	10 (1.9)	
No	527 (95.8)	25 (92.6)	502 (96.0)	
Experienced violence from community				.51
Yes	58 (10.6)	4 (14.8)	54 (10.3)	
No	491 (89.3)	23 (85.2)	468 (89.5)	
Has access to health services				.09
Yes	470 (85.5)	20 (74.1)	450 (86.0)	
No	80 (14.5)	7 (25.9)	73 (14.0)	
Has privacy where they live				.002
Yes	405 (73.6)	13 (48.2)	392 (75.0)	
No	144 (26.2)	14 (51.9)	130 (24.9)	
Feels in danger where they sleep				.22
Yes	129 (23.5)	9 (33.3)	120 (22.9)	
No	420 (76.4)	18 (66.7)	402 (76.9)	
Primary place of solicitation				.001
Street or public space	212 (38.6)	19 (70.4)	193 (36.9)	
Indoor establishment	139 (25.3)	1 (3.7)	138 (26.4)	
Independent	191 (34.7)	7 (25.9)	184 (35.2)	
Experienced police harassment				.1
Yes	51 (9.3)	5 (18.5)	46 (8.8)	
No	496 (90.2)	22 (81.5)	474 (90.6)	
Ever been incarcerated				.02
Yes	34 (6.2)	5 (18.5)	29 (5.5)	
No	516 (93.8)	22 (81.5)	494 (94.5)	
Monthly income, CAD	2260 (1280–4000)	2890 (1010–5840)	2205 (1280–3890)	.3

Note. CAD = Canadian dollars; IPV = intimate partner violence; IQR = interquartile range.

Our study provides some of the first rigorous prospective cohort data regarding the relationship between housing and violence among women sex workers. Our findings are consistent with previous research demonstrating a high prevalence of violence among precariously housed women.[27–29] Our findings provide new insights into the relationship between various indicators of housing precarity—housing instability and evictions—with physical and sexual violence across both intimate partner and occupational settings. These findings are particularly important, as rising gendered violence and housing precarity have become increasing concerns amid the COVID-19 pandemic.[30]

In Canada—as in other high-income contexts—many sex workers have been unable to access government benefits and supports afforded to other service workers during the pandemic,[31] and temporary moratoria on rental evictions ended in August 2020. Many sex workers in British Columbia further reside in housing settings that were not covered by these moratoria (e.g., emergency shelters, transitional or recovery housing, some single-room occupancy hotels, and accommodations shared with property owners), contributing to housing precarity. In addition, many buildings in which sex workers live and work in Vancouver implemented "no-guest" policies because of COVID-19 concerns, which may have forced women to work in more dangerous settings or lose their housing.

TABLE 3— Time-Updated Models of the Relationship Between Exposure to Housing Instability and Evictions and Violence Outcomes Among Women Sex Workers: Vancouver, Canada, 2010–2019

Primary Exposures	Outcomes	OR (95% CI)	AOR (95% CI)
Model 1			
Experienced unstable housing[a]	Experienced IPV[a]	1.74 (1.48, 2.03)	2.04 (1.45, 2.87)[b]
No unstable housing	No IPV	1 (Ref)	1 (Ref)
Model 2			
Experienced unstable housing[a]	Experienced workplace violence[a]	1.57 (1.37, 1.81)	1.46 (1.06, 2.00)[c]
No unstable housing	No workplace violence[a]	1 (Ref)	1 (Ref)
Model 3			
Experienced eviction[a]	Experienced IPV[a]	2.52 (1.35, 4.69)	2.45 (0.99, 6.07)[d]
No eviction	No IPV[a]	1 (Ref)	1 (Ref)

Note. AOR = adjusted odds ratio; CI = confidence interval; IPV = intimate partner violence; OR = odds ratio.
[a]Time-updated measure refers to occurrences in the past 6 months at each biannual study visit.
[b]Model 1 adjusted for childhood trauma; n = 612; 2010–2019.
[c]Model 2 adjusted for age, Indigenous status, injection drug use,[a] mental health diagnosis, childhood trauma, and place of solicitation[a]; n = 898; 2010–2019.
[d]Model 3 adjusted for age, childhood trauma, and average monthly income[a]; n = 273; 2014–2019.

Finally, women in our study who used both injection and noninjection drugs faced far higher proportions of unstable housing and evictions than those who did not use drugs. Previous work examining the relationship between housing and violence among women who use drugs has articulated the inadequacy of single-room occupancy hotels, which are among the most common affordable housing options for marginalized women who use substances in Vancouver.[32,33] More research is needed on harm-reduction housing strategies as a potential means to reduce IPV. The scale-up of programs that provide women who use substances with affordable, safe, and dignified housing options is urgently needed.

Limitations and Strengths

Our study has several limitations of note. There is potential for information bias resulting from the use of self-reported measures; to mitigate this, trained interviewers with lived experiences and strong personal connections to the community conducted outreach and administered surveys. In addition, our measure of IPV captured experiences of violence perpetuated by only male partners and did not address IPV by other perpetrators. Some effect sizes, particularly for analyses of exposure to evictions, may be a result of limited statistical power.

Our study also has several strengths. Our analysis provides a foundation for beginning to quantitatively understand the relationship between housing instability and gender-based violence among women sex workers. Future mixed-methods and path analyses may be beneficial to understand specific explanatory mechanisms underpinning the observed associations. Future research should also evaluate structural interventions to improve housing stability and safety among sex workers, as well as the impact of the COVID-19 pandemic on housing instability and gender-based violence among sex workers.

Policy and Practice Implications

There is a crucial need to address housing instability, evictions, and high rates of IPV and workplace violence experienced by sex workers, including youths, gender and sexual minorities, and Indigenous women. The high burden of housing instability and evictions documented in this study highlights the urgent need to decriminalize sex work to address barriers related to criminalization and stigma, which undermine sex workers' human rights related to housing. Decriminalization is a recognized best practice and evidence-based intervention for improving sex workers' health, safety, and human rights, which includes the right to an adequate standard of living.

Women-specific supportive housing options that meaningfully address sex workers' health and safety are also needed, for example, affordable, women-centered housing with flexible guest policies, security measures, community-based support staff, and integrated harm-reduction supports.[6,18,34] More broadly, scale-up of affordable housing options is needed for marginalized women, as research has shown that rising gentrification poses a high risk of disconnecting women from essential services.[35] In addition, the extension of government-implemented eviction moratoria could potentially mitigate the risk of gender-based violence for sex workers facing housing instability.

Conclusions

We have documented a high burden of unstable housing and evictions among women sex workers in Metro Vancouver. We found that exposure to unstable housing was associated with significantly higher odds of experiencing IPV and workplace violence over a 9-year observation period and that exposure to evictions was associated with elevated odds of IPV over a 4.5-year observation period. To support sex workers' occupational safety and human rights, public health interventions should include structural changes to scale up safe, affordable, and supportive housing for marginalized women as well as decriminalization of sex work to address housing barriers that are produced and reproduced by pervasive criminalization and stigma. AJPH

ABOUT THE AUTHORS

Shira M. Goldenberg is with the School of Public Health, San Diego State University, CA. Natalie Buglioni recently graduated from the Faculty of Health Sciences, Simon Fraser University, Burnaby, BC. Andrea Krüsi and Kate Shannon are with the Department of Medicine, University of British Columbia (UBC), Vancouver. Elizabeth Frost is a doctoral student in the Joint Doctoral Program in Public Health (Epidemiology), San Diego State University–University of California, San Diego. Sarah Moreheart is a doctoral student in the Faculty of Health Sciences, Simon Fraser University. Melissa Braschel is with the Centre for Gender & Sexual Health Equity, UBC.

CORRESPONDENCE

Correspondence should be sent to Shira M. Goldenberg, PhD, Assistant Professor, Division of Epidemiology and Biostatistics, School of Public Health, San Diego State University, 5500 Campanile Dr, San Diego, CA 92182-1308 (e-mail: dr.goldenberg@cgshe.ubc.ca). Reprints can be ordered at http://www.ajph.org by clicking the "Reprints" link.

PUBLICATION INFORMATION

Full Citation: Goldenberg SM, Buglioni N, Krüsi A, et al. Housing instability and evictions linked to elevated intimate partner and workplace violence among women sex workers in Vancouver, Canada: findings of a prospective, community-based cohort, 2010–2019. *Am J Public Health*. 2023;113(4): 442–452.

Acceptance Date: December 13, 2022.

DOI: https://doi.org/10.2105/AJPH.2022.307207

CONTRIBUTORS

S. M. Goldenberg and N. Buglioni conceptualized the study and wrote the article. S. M. Goldenberg, N. Buglioni, A. Krüsi, and M. Braschel interpreted the data. S. M. Goldenberg, N. Buglioni, and E. Frost performed the literature review. S. M. Goldenberg, A. Krüsi, E. Frost, S. Moreheart, and K. Shannon critically reviewed and revised the article. S. M. Goldenberg, S. Moreheart, and K. Shannon oversaw collection of the data. S. M. Goldenberg and K. Shannon acquired study funding. M. Braschel developed the statistical methods and analyzed the data.

ACKNOWLEDGMENTS

This research was supported by the US National Institutes of Health (NIH; grant R01DA028648) and the Canadian Institutes of Health Research. S. M. Goldenberg was partially supported by the NIH. N. Buglioni was partially supported by Mitacs. S. Moreheart was supported by a Simon Fraser University doctoral scholarship. K. Shannon was partially supported by a Canada Research Chair in Gender Equity, Sexual Health and Global Policy and the NIH.

We are tremendously grateful to all An Evaluation of Sex Workers Health Access (AESHA) participants for their valuable contributions of time and expertise to this research. We thank all those who contributed their time and expertise to this project, including AESHA community advisory board members and partner agencies and the AESHA team, including the following: Emma Ettinger, Christie Gabriel, Jennifer McDermid, Jennifer Morris, Emily Luo, Becca Norris, Alka Murphy, Natasha Feuchuk, Alex Martin, Jennie Pearson, Yinong Zhao, Amber Stefanson, Maddie Hibbs, Arveen Kaur, Peter Vann, and Preet Dhanda.

Note. The content of this article is solely the responsibility of the authors and does not necessarily represent the official views of the funders.

CONFLICTS OF INTEREST

The authors have no conflicts of interest to report.

HUMAN PARTICIPANT PROTECTION

The study received ethical approval from the Providence Health Care and University of British Columbia and Simon Fraser University research ethics boards. All participants provided written informed consent before participating in the study.

REFERENCES

1. Swope CB, Hernández D. Housing as a determinant of health equity: a conceptual model. *Soc Sci Med*. 2019;243:112571. https://doi.org/10.1016/j.socscimed.2019.112571
2. Shannon K, Crago AL, Baral SD, et al. The global response and unmet actions for HIV and sex workers. *Lancet*. 2018;392(10148):698–710. https://doi.org/10.1016/S0140-6736(18)31439-9.
3. Decker MR, Crago AL, Chu SKH, et al. Human rights violations against sex workers: burden and effect on HIV. *Lancet*. 2015;385(9963):186–199. doi: 10.1016/S0140-6736(14)60800-X
4. Deering KN, Amin A, Shoveller J, et al. A systematic review of the correlates of violence against sex workers. *Am J Public Health*. 2014;104(5):e42–e54. https://doi.org/10.2105/AJPH.2014.301909
5. Lyons T, Krüsi A, Edgar E, Machat S, Kerr T, Shannon K. The impacts of intersecting stigmas on health and housing experiences of queer women sex workers in Vancouver, Canada. *J Homosex*. 2021;68(6):957–972. https://doi.org/10.1080/00918369.2019.1694337
6. Lazarus L, Chettiar J, Deering K, Nabess R, Shannon K. Risky health environments: women sex workers' struggles to find safe, secure and non-exploitative housing in Canada's poorest postal code. *Soc Sci Med*. 2011;73(11):1600–1607. https://doi.org/10.1016/j.socscimed.2011.09.015
7. Sandoval-Olascoaga S, Venkataramani AS, Arcaya MC. Eviction moratoria expiration and COVID-19 infection risk across strata of health and socioeconomic status in the United States. *JAMA Netw Open*. 2021;4(8):e2129041. https://doi.org/10.1001/jamanetworkopen.2021.29041
8. Leifheit KM, Linton SL, Raifman J, et al. Expiring eviction moratoriums and COVID-19 incidence and mortality. *Am J Epidemiol*. 2021;190(12): 2503–2510. https://doi.org/10.1093/aje/kwab196
9. Pavao J, Alvarez J, Baumrind N, Induni M, Kimerling R. Intimate partner violence and housing instability. *Am J Prev Med*. 2007;32(2):143–146. https://doi.org/10.1016/j.amepre.2006.10.008
10. Gilroy H, McFarlane J, Maddoux J, Sullivan C. Homelessness, housing instability, intimate partner violence, mental health, and functioning: A multi-year cohort study of IPV survivors and their children. *J Soc Distress Homeless*. 2016;25(2):86–94. https://doi.org/10.1080/10530789.2016.1245258
11. Footer KHA, White RH, Park JN, Decker MR, Lutnick A, Sherman SG. Entry to sex trade and long-term vulnerabilities of female sex workers who enter the sex trade before the age of eighteen. *J Urban Health*. 2020;97(3):406–417. https://doi.org/10.1007/s11524-019-00410-z
12. Duff P, Deering K, Gibson K, Tyndall M, Shannon K. Homelessness among a cohort of women in street-based sex work: the need for safer environment interventions. *BMC Public Health*. 2011;11(1):643. https://doi.org/10.1186/1471-2458-11-643
13. Surratt HL, Inciardi JA. HIV risk, seropositivity and predictors of infection among homeless and non-homeless women sex workers in Miami, Florida, USA. *AIDS Care*. 2004;16(5):594–604. doi: 10.1080/09540120410001716397
14. Petry L, Hill C, Milburn N, Rice E. Who is couch-surfing and who is on the streets? Disparities among racial and sexual minority youth in experiences of homelessness. *J Adolesc Health*. 2022;70(5):743–750. https://doi.org/10.1016/j.jadohealth.2021.10.039

15. Hail-Jares K, Vichta-Ohlsen R, Nash C. Safer inside? Comparing the experiences and risks faced by young people who couch-surf and sleep rough. *J Youth Stud.* 2020;24(3):305–322. https://doi.org/10.1080/13676261.2020.1727425
16. Knight KR, Lopez AM, Comfort M, Shumway M, Cohen J, Riley ED. Single room occupancy (SRO) hotels as mental health risk environments among impoverished women: the intersection of policy, drug use, trauma, and urban space. *Int J Drug Policy.* 2014;25(3):556–561. https://doi.org/10.1016/j.drugpo.2013.10.011
17. Lyons T, Krüsi A, Pierre L, Smith A, Small W, Shannon K. Experiences of trans women and two-spirit persons accessing women-specific health and housing services in a downtown neighborhood of Vancouver, Canada. *LGBT Health.* 2016;3(5):373–378. https://doi.org/10.1089/lgbt.2016.0060
18. Krüsi A, Chettiar J, Ridgway A, Abbott J, Strathdee SA, Shannon K. Negotiating safety and sexual risk reduction with clients in unsanctioned safer indoor sex work environments: a qualitative study. *Am J Public Health.* 2012;102(6):1154–1159. https://doi.org/10.2105/AJPH.2011.300638
19. Reed E, Gupta J, Biradavolu M, Devireddy V, Blankenship KM. The role of housing in determining HIV risk among female sex workers in Andhra Pradesh, India: considering women's life contexts. *Soc Sci Med.* 2011;72(5):710–716. https://doi.org/10.1016/j.socscimed.2010.12.009
20. Katsulis Y, Durfee A, Lopez V, Robillard A. Predictors of workplace violence among female sex workers in Tijuana, Mexico. *Violence Against Women.* 2015;21(5):571–597. https://doi.org/10.1177/1077801214545283
21. Yakubovich AR, Bartsch A, Metheny N, Gesink D, O'Campo P. Housing interventions for women experiencing intimate partner violence: a systematic review. *Lancet Public Health.* 2022;7(1):e23–e35. https://doi.org/10.1016/S2468-2667(21)00234-6
22. Argento E, Muldoon KA, Duff P, Simo A, Deering KN, Shannon K. High prevalence and partner correlates of physical and sexual violence by intimate partners among street and off-street sex workers. *PLoS ONE.* 2014;9(7):e102129. https://doi.org/10.1371/journal.pone.0102129
23. Goldenberg SM, Liyanage R, Braschel M, Shannon K. Structural barriers to condom access in a community-based cohort of sex workers in Vancouver, Canada: influence of policing, violence, and end-demand criminalization. *BMJ Sex Reprod Health.* 2020;46(4):301–307. https://doi.org/10.1136/bmjsrh-2019-200408
24. Stueve A, O'Donnell LN, Duran R, San Doval A, Blome J. Time-space sampling in minority communities: results with young Latino men who have sex with men. *Am J Public Health.* 2001;91(6):922–926. https://doi.org/10.2105/ajph.91.6.922
25. Garcia-Moreno C, Jansen HAFM, Ellsberg M, Heise L, Watts C. *WHO Multi-Country Study on Women's Health and Domestic Violence Against Women: Initial Results on Prevalence, Health Outcomes and Women's Responses.* Geneva, Switzerland: World Health Organization; 2005.
26. Maldonado G, Greenland S. Simulation study of confounder-selection strategies. *Am J Epidemiol.* 1993;138(11):923–936. https://doi.org/10.1093/oxfordjournals.aje.a116813
27. Riley ED, Cohen J, Knight KR, Decker A, Marson K, Shumway M. Recent violence in a community-based sample of homeless and unstably housed women with high levels of psychiatric comorbidity. *Am J Public Health.* 2014;104(9):1657–1663. https://doi.org/10.2105/AJPH.2014.301958
28. Riley ED, Vittinghoff E, Kagawa RMC, et al. Violence and emergency department use among community-recruited women who experience homelessness and housing instability. *J Urban Health.* 2020;97(1):78–87. https://doi.org/10.1007/s11524-019-00404-x
29. Kennedy MC, McNeil R, Milloy MJ, Dong H, Kerr T, Hayashi K. Residential eviction and exposure to violence among people who inject drugs in Vancouver, Canada. *Int J Drug Policy.* 2017;41:59–64. https://doi.org/10.1016/j.drugpo.2016.12.017
30. Roesch E, Amin A, Gupta J, García-Moreno C. Violence against women during COVID-19 pandemic restrictions. *BMJ.* 2020;369:m1712. https://doi.org/10.1136/bmj.m1712
31. Pearson J, Shannon K, Krusi A, et al. Barriers to governmental income supports for sex workers during COVID-19: results of a community-based cohort in Metro Vancouver. Available at: https://www.mdpi.com/2076-0760/11/9/383. Accessed January 14, 2023.
32. Collins AB, Boyd J, Damon W, et al. Surviving the housing crisis: social violence and the production of evictions among women who use drugs in Vancouver, Canada. *Health Place.* 2018;51:174–181. https://doi.org/10.1016/j.healthplace.2018.04.001
33. Vancouver Coastal Health Authority. Women's health and safety in the downtown Eastside: companion paper to the second generation strategy design paper. October 2016. Available at: http://www.vch.ca/Documents/DTES-Womens-Companion-Paper.pdf. Accessed January 14, 2023.
34. Collins AB, Boyd J, Hayashi K, Cooper HLF, Goldenberg S, McNeil R. Women's utilization of housing-based overdose prevention sites in Vancouver, Canada: an ethnographic study. *Int J Drug Policy.* 2020;76:102641. https://doi.org/10.1016/j.drugpo.2019.102641
35. Goldenberg SM, Amram O, Braschel M, Moreheart S, Shannon K. Urban gentrification and declining access to HIV/STI, sexual health, and outreach services amongst women sex workers between 2010–2014: results of a community-based longitudinal cohort. *Health Place.* 2020;62:102288. https://doi.org/10.1016/j.healthplace.2020.102288

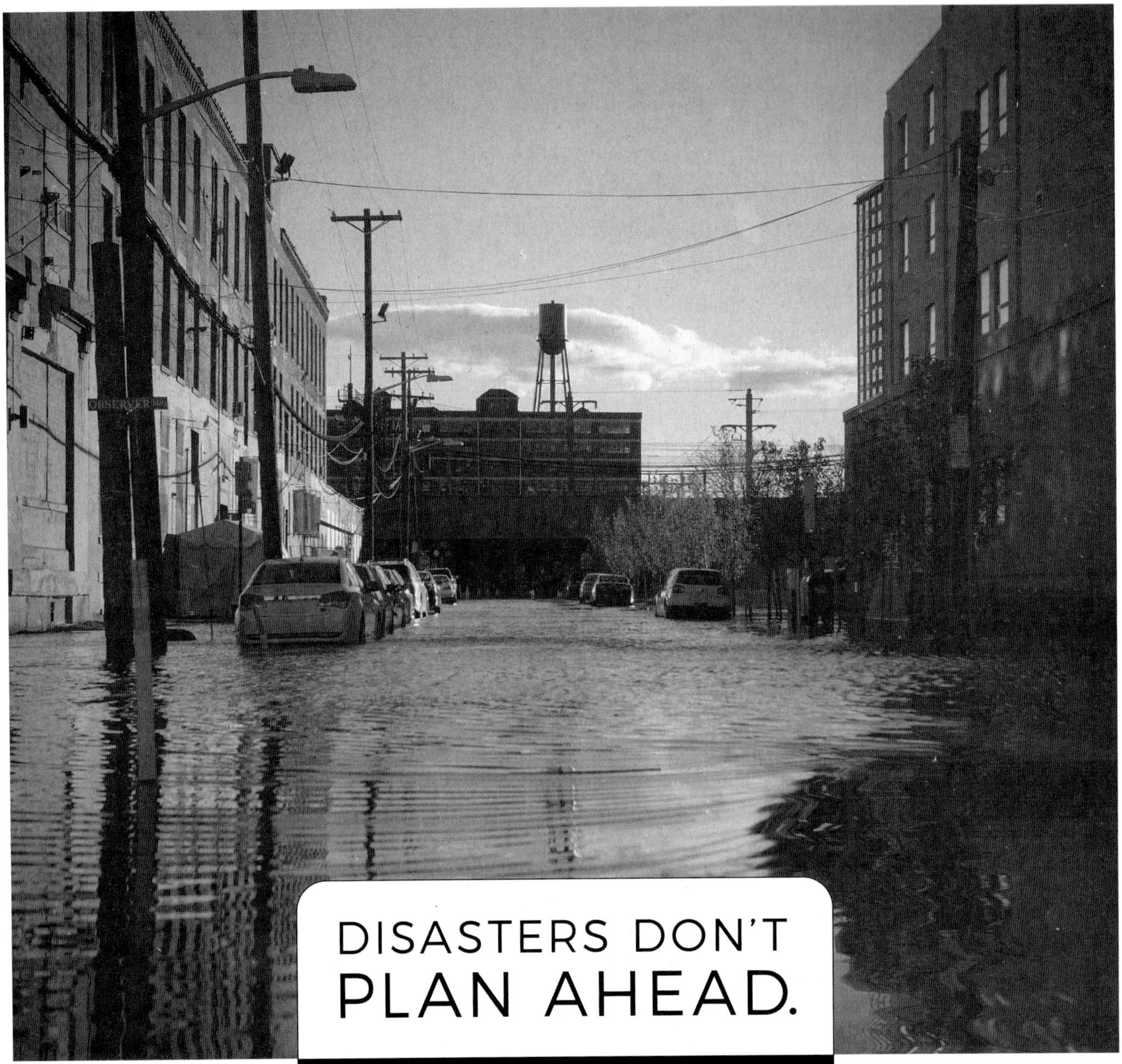

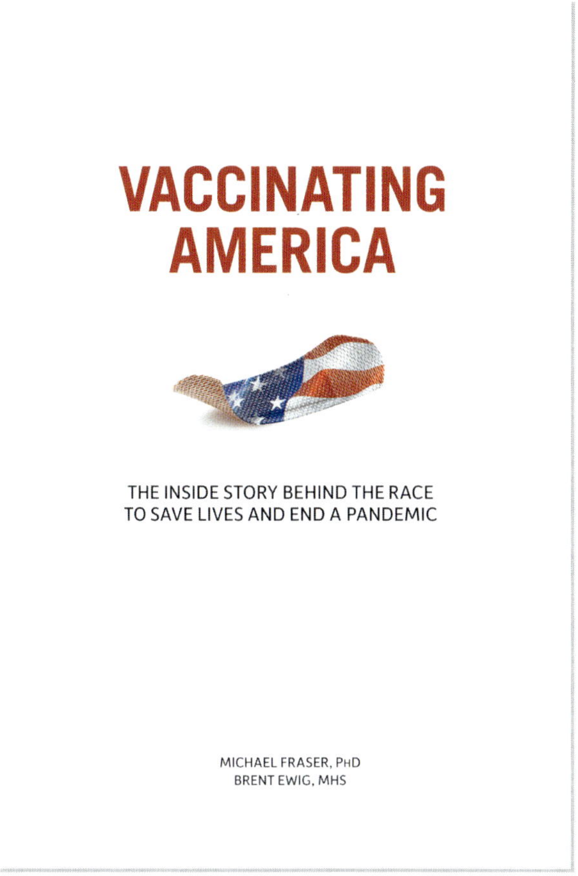

Vaccinating America: The Inside Story Behind the Race to Save Lives, and End a Pandemic

Edited by: Michael Fraser, PhD,
Brent Ewig, MHS

2023, 250 PP, SFTCVR, ISBN 978-0-87553-332-2

Vaccinating America spotlights the public servants and heroes who planned and executed this unprecedented program to combat COVID-19 amidst fierce partisan divides, bureaucratic infighting and overwhelming logistical challenges, and doesn't hold back on pointing out those who hindered progress.

APHABOOKSTORE.ORG

APHA PRESS

AN IMPRINT OF **AMERICAN PUBLIC HEALTH ASSOCIATION**

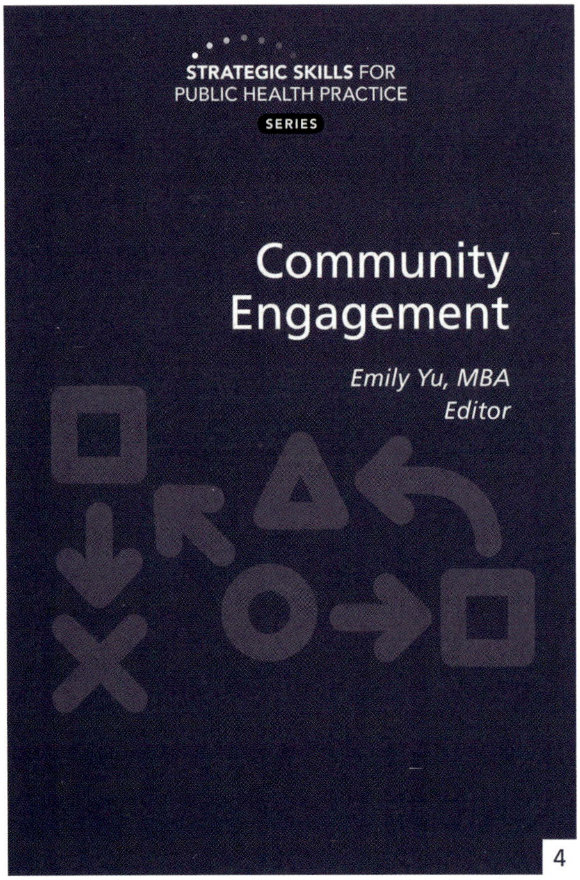

978-087553-3308, 108 PP, DIGITAL & SOFTCOVER

Community Engagement

Edited by Emily Yu, MBA

Community Engagement is the first book to be published from our new *Strategic Skills for Public Health Practice* series. This book brings the concept of community engagement to life through first-person stories, real-world examples and valuable insights from leaders across sectors. Curated specifically for public health practitioners and those interested in supporting community health, the book's chapters, guidance, and perspectives from the field will enhance readers' understanding of community-centered design and provide the tools to support organizational practices that drive better health for all.

APHABOOKSTORE.ORG

APHA PRESS

AN IMPRINT OF AMERICAN PUBLIC HEALTH ASSOCIATION